This Won't Hurt a Bit

This Won't Hurt a Bit
(and Other White Lies)

*My Education in Medicine
and Motherhood*

Michelle Au, MD

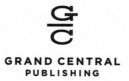

GRAND CENTRAL
PUBLISHING

NEW YORK   BOSTON

Copyright © 2011 by Michelle Au

Grand Central Publishing
Hachette Book Group
237 Park Avenue
New York, NY 10017

www.HachetteBookGroup.com

Printed in the United States of America

First Edition: May 2011

10 9 8 7 6 5 4 3 2 1

Grand Central Publishing is a division of Hachette Book Group, Inc.
The Grand Central Publishing name and logo is a trademark of Hachette Book Group, Inc.

Library of Congress Cataloging-in-Publication Data
Au, Michelle
   This won't hurt a bit: my education in medicine and motherhood / Michelle Au—1st ed.
      p. cm.
   Summary: "A hilarious and poignant memoir of a medical residency."—Provided by the publisher.
   ISBN 978-0-446-53824-4
   1. Au, Michelle. 2. Residents (Medicine)—United States—Biography. 3. Women physicians—United States—Biography. I. Title.
   [DNLM: 1. Au, Michelle. 2. Internship and Residency—methods—Personal Narratives. 3. Physicians, Women—Personal Narratives. WZ 100 A8875w 2011]
   R134.A9 2011
   610.92—dc22
                                        2010019040

To Joe, with much love.

Also to Cal and Mack, without whom life would be 50 percent more convenient but 100 percent less fun.

CONTENTS

This Won't Hurt a Bit

1 . APOLOGIA

WHAT IS HAPPENING NOW IS THIS: I am wearing a pair of too-large latex gloves, with my right hand reaching up between an eighty-five-year-old man's legs, searching for his anus.

He is a large man, more than 300 pounds, and extremely demented, flanked on one side by my intern and on the other by his nurse, who are both struggling, holding his legs apart to aid me in the hunt. My goal is to stick my index finger into his rectum and retrieve a piece of stool, so that I might smear said stool on a guaiac card to check for occult bleeding in his gastrointestinal tract.

But I am not thinking about occult bleeding in the gastrointestinal tract, or this patient, or his multiple medical problems, or his anxious wife hovering outside, one ear to the door, listening to everything. What I am thinking about is how it is now 5:00 p.m. and I still haven't eaten lunch, and how right after the ritual smearing-of-card-with-poop, I will be making a beeline to the nursing station, where I think I saw a few stale bagels laid out, left over from Grand Rounds this morning. *I am going to eat those bagels,* I think with a grim determination as I insinuate my gloved hand into a fold.

"Help me!" the patient screams. "They're stealing my money!"

"IT'S OK, MR. MOSKOWITZ, WE'RE JUST DOING A QUICK TEST, WE'LL BE FINISHED SOON," the resident bellows, in that tone of false, gritted-teeth cheer completely familiar to anyone who has spent any time at all in a hospital. I am a third-year medical student, and this is my General Surgery rotation. Despite the rosy notions with which I started my medical training—that even as a medical student I would be Helping People and Making a Difference and perhaps showcasing my flawless diagnostic acumen honed after two years in front of textbooks, making neat but never showy saves while my overtired resident sat oblivious in the corner with a pile of charts—what I had come to learn over the last year was that in the world of academic medicine, students are viewed as being good for only three things: writing long, overly detailed notes in the charts that no one, save other medical students, will ever read; changing CDs on the operating room stereo while the surgeons are scrubbed into a case; and doing the menial dirty work that no resident would ever do if he or she could find some way to avoid it.

"Help me! Help! Aaaah!" Mr. Moskowitz is still screaming. I wonder what this must sound like to his roommate, who is cowering silently on the other side of the pulled curtain.

"Did you get it yet?" My resident looks sweaty and harassed, holding up Mr. Moskowitz's legs, trying to clear a path of flesh enough for me to get where I need to go. I can read his face and see that he is thinking about the other twenty-three patients on his list and all the things he needs to do before he can sign them out to the overnight resident and go home. His pager goes off again, the second time since we've been in the room.

"Umm, almost." Not wanting to be branded as the med student who couldn't even find a patient's asshole, I don't have the heart to tell him that I'm not even close. Gingerly, with my left hand, I lift up Mr. Moskowitz's scrotum, figuring that whatever crack lies in the middle underneath is most probably my best bet. I find what looks like a promising track and, with my gloved hand, start to work my way backward within the fold.

"Did you Surgilube up?" My resident is starting to look the way I feel—like he wishes that he were dead.

"Surgilube? Uh...no, I forgot." Silently, but with perhaps as much contempt as one can express without saying a word, the nurse rips open a pack of water-soluble lubricant and squirts a dollop onto a piece of dry gauze. I reach up, almost losing my glove in the process, and coat my right index finger with the gloppy clear goo. "Thanks." The nurse just exhales forcefully through her nose.

"Now go for it," my resident says to me. To the

patient, about twenty decibels louder, he adds, "OK NOW, ALMOST DONE! JUST ANOTHER SECOND!" Perhaps as an indictment of my skill, Mr. Moskowitz gazes off into middle distance and farts.

"OK, I just need a little bit longer." I follow the same fold of skin backward, figuring that at some point I will hit a puckered hiatus, reach in, hit pay dirt, and end this nightmare for all of us. I move posteriorly, more, and then some more, until my hand is down against the bed. Nothing but a dead end. How could there be nothing there? Is it possible he doesn't *have* an anus?

"What can we do to help?" my resident asks in a tone of voice that leaves no question: *finish this thing or I am going to kill you.*

"Maybe...maybe lift him up a little more?" Grunting and straining, the resident and nurse manage to roll Mr. Moskowitz's butt up a few more inches. Reaching back farther, sweaty and hungry and desperate for a chance to wash my hands, I finally feel what I'm looking for. Poking one lubed finger through, I find a piece of stool perilously close to the surface, and with a small hooking motion, scrape off a small piece and pull out my hand. Panting, I look at my gloved finger with the small piece of fecal matter balancing on the tip and feel absurdly pleased.

My resident is already snapping off his gloves and heading out of the room. "Let me know if it's positive," he says as he's walking out the door—to the patient's wife, waiting outside, he shouts, slowing down but not stopping, "HE DID GREAT, WE SHOULD

HAVE THOSE RESULTS IN JUST A FEW MINUTES, OK?" And then he's gone.

I'm still standing there with my brown-tinged finger. "Wait, now what do I do?" The nurse silently hands me the card and the bottle of developer. I scrape some of the stool onto the little windows on the front of the card and drip on some of the clear developer fluid. If the test is positive for blood, the fluid around the stool should turn a grayish blue after three minutes. If it's negative for blood, there will be no color change. I take the card, stick it into a clean glove, and then put the whole package into my pocket, figuring I will check it again once three minutes has elapsed. "Mr. Moskowitz, the test is finished. I'm sorry if it was unpleasant," I say as I pull down his hospital gown and replace the bedsheet over his chest.

"They stole everything from me, you know," he says conversationally. Then, as if it's somehow related, he adds, "You're a good girl." I guess all is forgiven.

I wash my hands and walk back to the nursing station, where I find that someone has already eaten the rest of the day-old bagels. I rescue a few stray poppy seeds and stick them in my mouth morosely, feeling like Oliver Twist, almost relishing this pathetic tableau. Just then, I see my boyfriend, Joe, a fellow medical student rotating through the Vascular Surgery service while I'm on Colorectal. "How's it going?" he asks.

"Shitty. It just took me about half an hour to guaiac some guy because I couldn't find his asshole."

He makes a sympathetic noise. "Don't feel bad.

My resident just told Andy and me to Foley some lady" (that is, to insert a Foley catheter into her urethra to drain the bladder) "and Andy accidentally tried to catheterize her clitoris."

I made a pained face. "Hmm. But actually, that *does* make me feel better." Joe makes a *see you later* gesture before walking away, and I pull out the guaiac card from the glove in my pocket to check on the results. The test window is a light grayish color. While it is clear that a deep grayish blue would be Bad and no color change would be Good, I really don't know what to make of the light gray. As if on cue, my pager goes off. It's my resident.

"So what did the guaiac show?" he asks when I call him back. The noise in the background sounds like he's at another nursing station, and I hear voices, as if he's simultaneously having another conversation while on the phone with me. "Yeah. No, the other guy with the perf. Tomorrow." And then a little louder, into the receiver, "Was it positive?"

"Uh, the guaiac? Um...see..." I'm not really sure what to tell him. "I think it *could* be positive, but it's not, like, *so* positive. Like, instead of really dark blue, it's only tinted light gray, but it's not, you know, *nothing*. So I can't really say that it's negative either. It's sort of...so-so."

There is a silence. "I'll come by and take a look." And with an aggrieved sigh and some unintelligible mutter, he hangs up. I wonder if I am the stupidest medical student he's ever worked with. I wonder if I am the stupidest medical student in the class. I wonder if it's possible to get kicked out of medical school for being unable to interpret the results of a stool guaiac. And now the nurse is yelling at me because I accidentally left the guaiac card with its hard-won brown smears on the table next to the empty bagel tray, and people *eat* at this table, don't you even know you shouldn't be bringing patient samples back behind the desk, what in the hell is *wrong* with you?

Scutmonkey

Why do people decide to become doctors anyway?

Let's look at this first purely from the perspective of personal investment and expectation. To practice medicine, first, you have to go to medical school. That's four years right there. Then, there's residency, which adds anywhere between three and seven years to the deal. After that, there may be a fellowship, sometimes two fellowships, because really, at that point, what's another year or two (or six)? So basically, from the moment you start into medical school to the moment you finish your training, you're looking at *a minimum* of seven years—for most people it's closer to ten—before you're even close to being considered a "real" doctor.

And these are not fun, carefree years—certainly not the way most people spend their twenties, at least if the producers of MTV or beer advertisers are to be believed. You spend these fetal-doctor years indoors under fluorescent lighting, nose pressed into books filled with inscrutable diagrams and endless acronyms, while everyone in the world, including some of your patients, appears to be having more fun than you. These are years spent doing a whole lot of work for little or no money, ignominious tasks relegated to those contractually obligated to never complain. These are years of thousands of lost hours spent at the hospital instead of with your friends and family, who always seem to be wondering where you are and why you're still there and when, if ever, you'll be coming home. These are years spent defying all common sense about circadian rhythms and the regenerative powers of rest, largely awake and caffeinated to an almost toxic degree. And—this last part is the real kicker—these are years after which you will end up in hundreds and thousands of dollars of debt, all for the experience of what amounts to hard time in a well-intentioned Soviet gulag. I repeat: *not fun.*

It was true that I wanted to be a doctor, but there were *other* things I wanted to be at the same time. Like many people I knew, I imagined that by the time I was thirty (OK, maybe thirty-five), I would be in a committed relationship with someone that I loved, or at least sort of liked. Maybe I would be married. Perhaps I would have kids, presented the time and the opportunity and provided that the corrosive powers of time did not rob me completely of my reproductive potential by the time I was ready for the responsibility. Barring that, maybe I would have a dog. Or at least a fish.

But then I would go into the hospital on my General Surgery rotation and see a bunch of bitter, tired men in their thirties, still years away from their first paying job, all either single or divorced or in some way separated from their spouses, and their sole message of wisdom to impart to their medical students was, *Dude, whatever you decide to do with your life, don't do* this.

But despite it all, despite the complete disconnect between the life of medicine as we saw it and the real life we envisioned for ourselves, many of us decided to become doctors anyway. Why? I believe that for most people, there's a spectrum of reasons.

First and hopefully underlying all the other reasons, there's probably the pure and honest desire to want to do good in life. *I want to help people.* Put aside the fact that many jobs are expressly designed to help people—the barista helps people by getting them their coffee, the dry cleaner helps people by pressing their shirts, the street mime helps people by making them realize that no matter how terrible they think their lives are, at least they're not street mimes—and you have what seems like a pretty good blanket answer to throw out there at interviews and family functions, provided that there are absolutely no follow-up questions. (Unfortunately, there always are.)

Perhaps some people have a special facility for applied science. That seems reasonable enough. There's so much Biology and Chemistry and Physics and Physiology in medicine that in medical school, we spend two straight years studying nothing else. That said, there are plenty of people who are gifted in Biology and Chemistry and Physics who have no business being anywhere near other human beings, and would perhaps better serve the world in the back of a computer lab, writing *Battlestar Galactica* fan fiction and engaging in heated online arguments with others doing the same.

Maybe you have had a Medical Experience, and as a result of your Medical Experience you had an epiphany and decided that you would like to become a doctor yourself. A personal incident of illness or injury, time spent caring for a sick parent, a particularly moving episode of *ER* circa The Clooney Years—this overall seems like a valid precursor to a career in medicine. (Well, maybe not the *ER* thing.) You have had an encounter in the field and have some true and earnest desire to either perpetuate the good that you have witnessed or to expose and eradicate the wrongs. However, if this were the main reason that people decided to become doctors, medical schools would be filled with classes of students with dead parents and crippled siblings, and at least from my experience, this is not overwhelmingly the case.

There *are*, however, plenty of people in medical school who have a doctor in the family. Usually one parent, sometimes both. Coming from a medical dynasty can have its pluses and minuses—on one hand, these people are usually down-to-earth and diligent, as they are going into the family business and know both what to expect and what is expected of them. On the other hand, some of them act like by virtue of birthright, they are doctors already, and the actual process of medical training is just an unfortunate technicality.

Sometimes people become doctors because it's a

well-respected field with which most people have a passing familiarity. The window dressings of medicine are well known to any layman with a television—the long white coats, the stethoscopes slung casually around the neck in battle-ready position, the Hippocratic oath to "first, do no harm." The doctor is an icon, instantly recognizable. Children tell parents they want to become doctors the same way they say they want to be teachers or scientists or astronauts, because they know what doctors are, and what they do, and because expressing an interest in medicine makes parents instantly happy. (Maybe there are some children who express the desire to be hedge fund managers when they grow up, but those children should probably be checked periodically for clustered sixes in the hairline.) Early on in medical school, some guys in my class used to go out to bars wearing their medical school IDs with the notion that it would help them pick up women. While their technique was dubious, they perhaps more than any of us understood the power and respect of the medical degree. And the thrill that a new intern feels the first time she is referred to as "Doctor" is universal and undeniable, the excitement of finally being accepted into an exclusive pantheon, something like being knighted.

And let's not beat around the bush, sometimes people decide to become doctors because of the money. No one talks about it, but risking excommunication, I'm telling you. It's hardly a "get rich quick" scheme, but for most of us, it is at least a "get moderately well-off slow" scheme. While I certainly don't think that you should go into medicine *solely* for the money (there are much easier ways to earn money—growing and selling your hair for high-end wigs comes to mind), I also don't think it's *wrong* to consider a career in medicine for its practical benefits. A stable career with good earning potential—isn't that what most people look for? But no, we don't speak of such earthly concerns, especially not when the popular notion of The Good Doctor imagines him subsisting solely on handshakes and goodwill. Though no one ever seems to want to talk about the details, I can confidently tell you that while income varies across specialties and geography, overall, doctors make a lot of money.

So there is altruism. There is the academic interest. There are societal influences and personal influences and there is of course the matter of money. Students going into medicine probably cycle through most if not all of these reasons at some point in their decision process, sometimes multiple times in one day. It is easier, for example, to be altruistic at 9:00 a.m. than at 2:00 a.m. Motivations also may change as an individual matures, and the rosy idealism of the twenty-two-year-old first-year med student may eventually give way to the real-world considerations of a married father of two trying to support a young family on a single salary. I can't understand everyone's reasons or the factors that temper their decisions, but in most cases it boils down to this: *we want to become good doctors because we want to be able to make a positive and meaningful difference in the lives of people when they need help the most.* And for this privilege, we're willing to deal with the rest of it.

But I will tell you one thing I know for certain. No one decides that they want to be a doctor because they want to be a scutmonkey.

* * *

So what, the civilians want to know, *is a scutmonkey?*

There are versions of scutmonkeys in most professions. The entertainment business has its production assistants, the mob has its "button men," and in medicine, we have our scutmonkeys—the hungry, scrabbling masses charged to do the jobs no one else wants. Sometimes these jobs are distasteful, almost always these jobs are menial, and not infrequently, these jobs are just flat-out *boring,* which is probably why *SCUT* is perhaps best understood as an acronym one of my residents passed on to me: "Sub-Cerebral Use of Time." And yet all of us in medicine, from the silver-haired senior attending on down, have at one time or another been scutmonkeys.

Luckily, being a scutmonkey is a temporary condition. It starts with medical school under the guise of education, fully manifests during residency and fellowship, when we are technically *paid* to get scutted out (and why senior doctors feel free to assign scutwork with much less guilt), and resolves itself fully upon completion of training. Despite the painful and often protracted nature of the scutmonkey years, senior doctors often seem to have a degree of retrograde amnesia when it comes to the travails it took to get them there. Sure, they have their stock of old war stories, which are pulled out, dusted off, and, like baby pictures, passed around the assembled audience, where they are duly admired or subversively one-upped. But overall, doctors finished with their training see themselves plucked from the mire and deposited into an altogether more agreeable lifestyle, not unlike Willis and Arnold on *Diff'rent Strokes*, though perhaps with even less interest in looking back. And really, it doesn't take long to forget the old neighborhood. "Honestly, things are *completely* different now," one young attending once told me. "It's *so* much better. You just wait and see. I can hardly *remember* what it was like to be a resident anymore. I honestly can't believe I used to *live* like that." She had graduated from her Pediatrics residency all of six months earlier.

Nobody goes into medicine to be a scutmonkey, but almost all of us look forward to what comes after. The day when, we envision, we will be able to practice medicine the way we want. The day when we will be able to decide *what* and *when* and *how* things will be done for our own patients during the day, and yet have enough freedom to have lives outside of the hospital as well. When we will be valued for our years of advanced education, for our clinical expertise, for our judgment, not just for the decerebrate ability to write down lab values and page EKG technicians and push stretchers from Point A to Point B at 3:00 a.m. The day when we will have scores of little scutmonkeys of our own to dispatch on a whim, to take care of the things that we will be too important to do.

But first, before we get to that point, we all have to pay our dues.

* * *

It is now almost nine at night, and I have somehow gotten roped into scrubbing into a bowel resection with Dr. Mareman. Dr. Mareman is a surgical attending with a slow, plodding operative style, the result of which is that routine cases sometimes last hours longer than expected, sessions groaningly referred to as "Mare-athons." I don't know *why* I am scrubbed into this case—I don't seem to be doing anything in the OR except consuming oxygen and taking up space that probably could better be used by someone who actually knows what they are doing—and yet I stand there, resplendently sterile in cap and gown and mask and feeling itchy.

Actually, I *do* know why I am scrubbed in. I am scrubbed because as I was leaving the hospital for the day, my senior resident grabbed me and said, "We need you to scrub into the Mare-athon in Room Five," and despite the fact that the reason for my presence was not clear, and that I am not on call that night, not to mention that I have a big presentation to give the following morning for which I have done almost no preparation, I don't say anything, because medical students aren't supposed to say no. Which is why for the last two hours, I have been standing next to the patient with my gloves held above my waist, resting them lightly on the sterile drapes as I have been instructed, trying not to contaminate myself.

"We've got to take down all these adhesions!" Dr. Mareman is instructing the resident scrubbed across the table from him. "These adhesions! We have! To take them down! How's his pressure? How are we doing? Do we need to transfuse? Is he OK?" Dr. Mareman is, to put it politely, spazzing out.

"He's doing fine. One twenties over eighties." The disembodied voice of the anesthesiologist floats serenely over the blue drape by the patient's head.

"Fine? OK. Good. Go. Let's go!" The senior resident's face is mostly obscured behind his surgical mask, but he sighs with his eyes. My own eyes flick to the clock again: *9:05.*

"Bovie this." Dr. Mareman indicates to the resident, who picks up the cauterizing surgical blade and cuts through a translucent plane of tissue. "This! This! Here, where my finger is!" I am standing alongside, completely peripheral to the action, not even holding an instrument or retracting skin from the surgical field. *I'm hungry,* I think.

"Look at this. This guy's a mess. How long has he been open?" This patient has been sitting on the surgical ward for weeks after multiple bowel surgeries, his abdomen left open for easy access, covered with a synthetic mesh sewn crudely to the skin. The last time I saw him, prior to this latest trip to the OR, he was lying in bed, his abdomen wrapped with an abdominal binder, naked except for his underwear, afraid to move for fear of disrupting the cacophony of tubing and monitoring surrounding him. "*Hola,*

Señor Cuevas," I ventured tentatively, basically exhausting my knowledge of medical Spanish with one sentence: "*Cómo se siente?*"

He groaned weakly. "*Aye, Dios.*" He gestured weakly to his abdomen, his emaciated body, the beeping IV pump, and the miles and miles of plastic tubing. "*Ayúdeme.*" He looked defeated. "*Ayúdeme.*"

I wanted to help him, of course, but I couldn't quite think of how. I couldn't even *talk* to him, as my Spanish skills don't allow me to say much more than "*Todo esta bien,*" but anyone with eyes and half a brain could look into this room and see that *todo* extremely *no esta bien.* Looking at his chart and his medication list and his splayed-open bowels, packed with gauze already turning greenish and malodorous from *Pseudomonas aeruginosa* bacteria, I felt just as hopeless as he, and barely able to do anything about it. Who was *I*, anyway? Not a surgeon who could close his wound, an infectious disease specialist who could analyze the sensitivities of the microbes growing out of every orifice of his body, or a psychiatrist who could help him deal with his crippling depression. I am none of these things. I'm just a medical student.

Back in the OR, Dr. Mareman is gesturing toward a length of bowel that looks dusky and strangulated. "Take this down here, and we'll clamp this off over on this side." He calls for the tools he needs, and he and the senior resident get to work, talking in shorthand, mumbling so softly that I can barely hear them. I don't think they even remember that I'm standing there.

Why am I here? I think to myself. *I'm useless. In fact, I might actually be compromising patient care. They could have a real doctor standing in my spot instead, someone who might actually have something useful to contribute to this surgery.* Then, changing tracks, I think, *I have to go to the bathroom. What do people do when they're scrubbed into those really long cases? When surgeons do a liver transplant, do they just wear those adult diapers? Or do they stick in a catheter at the start of the case and wear a leg bag?* I want to ask Dr. Mareman and the resident about the anatomy I'm seeing in front of me, and what blood supply they're isolating, but they look like they're concentrating hard and I don't want to interrupt them.

"Specimen," Dr. Mareman intones grandly, and a stapled length of bowel leaves Mr. Cuevas's abdomen and plops into a specimen bucket, where it is passed off to the circulating nurse to label for pathology. "Let's just check this again, and maybe we can try to close him." Instruments are removed, and the resident starts to run his finger through the lengths of bowel, which are pulsating feebly.

My nose itches. I look around furtively. *Man, why did they make me scrub into this case? Just to stand here? Is there a way for me to scratch my nose without compromising my sterility?* My surgical mask is sliding down, tickling my face, which only makes things worse. *I saw a surgical attending once ask the circulating nurse to scratch his forehead, but I very well couldn't do that, could I? She would get mad. I don't think medical students are allowed to itch. What if I'm allergic to latex?* The very thought makes me itch even more. I concentrate on the surgery in front of me, trying to keep my mind off the itching and the peeing and my rioting stomach, which last took in two saltine crackers and a Jell-O cup from a discarded patient tray four hours ago. *Actually, it wasn't even a Jell-O cup. It was a Gel Treat brand strawberry-flavored gelatin snack.*

Suddenly, on the field, I see a flash of bright green, like a spurt. Then again, a little winking jet of lime. There's a very small hole in the bowel. An accidental nick in the jejunum. Or maybe it's the ileum, I'm not really sure. It all happens quickly but I'm sure I saw correctly, and when no one else seems to notice, I have to speak up. "There's a hole," I say, my voice a little hoarse from three hours of keeping silent.

"What's that now?" the senior resident asks without looking up.

"There's a hole. I saw a hole. Just a tiny nick, but there was bilious fluid coming out." The words are coming faster now that I've gotten warmed up.

"Where?" Dr. Mareman, the resident, and I stare into the cavern of Mr. Cuevas's abdominal cavity. The small bowel sits there, looking innocent, and the small hole I saw just a moment ago is gone, possibly buried from view by the small peristaltic movements that look like a can of earthworms I once saw at a bait shop.

"There's no hole." The resident gets back to work, determined to finish up. It is past ten o'clock at this point.

"I think...I think there was. I saw something." I

19

don't want him to think that I'm accusing him of actually making the hole, right in front of the attending surgeon no less, so I try to shift the focus a little. "It's just...this guy has had a hard time. If we're going to close," (and oh, the conceit of that "we"!) "I just don't want him to have another leak and more problems down the line." The euphemism "problems" is perhaps understating things mildly. A bowel leak would basically entail liquid stool pouring from the patient's intestines into his abdominal cavity, leading to infection, abscess formation, sepsis, and death. In fact, a bowel leak was what originally brought Mr. Cuevas into our care several weeks ago. All three of us stare intently at the surgical field. There is no hole that any of us can see.

"Oh, medical student." The resident does not seem particularly upset, and he says this last with a sort of indulgent affection, despite the fact that he clearly has no idea what my name is. "Always looking out. I don't see a hole, though." Dr. Mareman asks for an instrument, and they resume the closure. I know what I saw, but I decide not to say anything more for now.

About thirty seconds later, very quickly, I see that bright green flash again. This time, I do not hesitate, but actually take my gloved hands off the drapes, reach toward the patient's bowels, and point. "There. That's what I saw. Right there." The resident grabs the bowel itself, and sure enough, there is a small hole. Another flick of peristalsis squirts a plume of bilious fluid out of the hole as Dr. Mareman peers down.

"Medical student! Eagle eye!" Dr. Mareman, instead of reacting with anger or annoyance as I had feared, seems delighted. The resident calls for a suture, and one small stitch is enough to hold the small hole closed. After satisfying themselves that the closure will hold, they resume closing the overlying tissue, then the skin. Forty-five minutes later, Mr. Cuevas's scarred abdomen is held shut by staples, he awakens from general anesthesia, and the anesthesia resident pulls his breathing tube as the patient gasps and coughs.

As the team readies Mr. Cuevas for transport to the recovery room, the surgical resident calls out to me, "Would you mind getting the music and bringing it back to the office for us?" Pulling off my gown and gloves, I walk over to the table where the small portable stereo sits, unplug it from the wall, and grab the stack of CDs sitting alongside it. Then, carrying this stash, I trot alongside Mr. Cuevas's stretcher, which is being wheeled out of the room. He is still groggy from the anesthesia, lying with his eyes closed, breathing supplemental oxygen through the clear tubing in his nose.

"*Señor Cuevas*," I say, and he opens his eyes confusedly. I don't know if he knows where he is, or what exactly just happened, but I want to tell him that his abdomen has been closed, hopefully for the last time. I scour my brain for the words to tell him. Finally I just say, "*Todo esta bien.*"

He nods slightly, and closes his eyes again. The stretcher is pushed faster, down the hall, and I am left behind, holding the stereo and a pile of CDs in cracked jewel boxes. It is late in the evening, and most of the ORs have finished up for the day, but even as I stand there, I see nurses and techs setting up another room for an emergency case yet to start. They rush past me in a flurry of blue, sneakers and clogs squeaking.

I return the music to the surgery office, being careful to stack the CDs neatly so that they don't fall on the floor. As I close the door to the office, I see that it is now 11:30 p.m., and I still have to finish my presentation for the next day before going to bed. I am due in at 3:45 the following morning to round on the patients on the Colorectal Surgery service. Mr. Cuevas will be out of the post-anesthesia care unit and back in his room by then, so I'll see him there.

As I walk through the hospital lobby on my way home, I feel a little less tired. "Goodnight, Doc," the security guard at the desk calls out to me. He says this to me often. Usually I am embarrassed when he does, the way he calls me "Doc" so casually. *I'm not a doctor,* I always think. *I don't deserve the title yet. I'm just a medical student. I just come here and learn and do what I'm told and try not to get in the way.*

But tonight, for the first time, I don't think these things. "Goodnight," I reply, "see you in a few hours." And I do.

2 . PRECLINICAL

Premedical

THE SPRING OF MY SENIOR YEAR of college, I read the book *Doctors* by Erich Segal. It was light, beach-type reading, which suited me at the time— given the choice, I wouldn't have engaged in any activity more intellectually strenuous than staring at my calendar willing the eight weeks until graduation to pass more quickly. The book was on loan from my roommate, who apologized in advance for its cheesiness, but told me that it was absorbing nonetheless and that I might enjoy the preview, since I was starting medical school in the fall.

I read the entire book in twenty-four hours. And my roommate was right—it *was* cheesy. But it had all the elements of a good medical story, fictional or not. Tragedy, triumph, ethical quandaries, hope, and redemption. The characters were a little two-dimensional, the plot creaky and predictable, but I devoured it, and despite mocking some of its more romantic flourishes, a small part of me bought the story completely.

I especially recall a scene early in the book when the dean addresses the class of first-year medical students for the first time. "Look to the left of you. Look to the right of you. One of the three of you will not make it to graduation." But oh, to be that one person of the three! The mortification! All those wasted years! How does one bounce back from such a blow? (Law school, perhaps.)

I grew up in a family of doctors. My parents were both doctors—having met in medical school and graduated in the hazy crazy era of 1970s New York City—completing their training in the rough-and-tumble inner-city hospitals of Upper Manhattan and the Bronx back when the streets were grimier, no one dared to walk near Central Park after dusk, and AIDS was still a looming shadow on the horizon. I grew up looking at pictures of my parents in medical school, grainy yellowing snapshots of their class posed stiffly at graduation, flanking the bust of Albert Einstein gracing the campus of the physicist's eponymous medical school in the Bronx, and wondering who in the world would ever trust a bunch of doctors who walked around looking like *that*, with their huge collars and bushy hair, clad in sickly brown, upholstery-looking fabrics.

Contrary to the stereotype of Chinese parents, my parents never encouraged me to go into medicine.

In fact, there were points throughout my childhood when they (my father in particular) actively tried to *dissuade* me from following in their footsteps, citing the increasing bureaucracy of medicine, the growing culture of litigation in American society that pushed more and more doctors to practice defensive, rather than sound, medicine, and of course, concerns for my safety. "If you have to be a doctor," my father once told me, in the mid-1980s, "at least go practice out in some small town somewhere in the mountains," where, the unspoken pretext was, I wouldn't be as likely to contract a deadly disease from my own patients or be shot in the head. (It is not clear that my father had ever actually *been* to any small towns in the mountains, but I think he had in mind a generally wholesome atmosphere, where patients came in to the hospital with, say, cowpox or a concussion after a tractor collision, rather than multiple knife wounds and hepatitis C from years of intravenous drug abuse.)

However, perhaps it was my own form of childhood rebellion (if so, the most halfhearted attempt at rebellion on record) that made me decide at a very young age to be a doctor. Because despite their protestations to the contrary, it was clear that my parents loved the work they did. They found it intellectually stimulating and emotionally gratifying, and when I was growing up, they worked long hours, six days a week, without complaint. I had only the vaguest idea of what it was that my parents actually *did* as doctors (my mother is a pediatric ophthalmologist and my father is a dermatologist; thus I spent much of my youth under the impression that my mother handed out glasses and my father put Band-Aids on people), but I had been to their offices several times, noted the equipment and the smells and the way their patients waited dutifully in the waiting room for their turn to be seen, and I always came away deeply impressed. Anyway, what child *really* knows what they want to be when they grow up anyway? Teacher, fireman, doctor, astronaut. Take your pick.

Moving past high school and through college, I got a clearer sense that becoming a doctor was not something that you simply *decided* to do, but rather something that required you to jump through certain hoops and work hard toward, and as such I had done my due diligence. I stacked my transcript with good grades in science and math, padded my resume with plenty of volunteer work, and spent six months in college in a neuroscience lab doing bench research (which I hated) because I thought that at least *some* effort to vivisect mice was an unspoken prerequisite for medical training. (For the record: it is not.) I sent in my applications to medical school the summer of 1998, applying widely but concentrating in the Northeast, particularly in New York. When I started getting acceptance letters, I hardly knew what to do. For years, I had worked toward the goal of being accepted into medical school, and now that I *had* been, I suddenly realized that I had no idea what came next. It was like finishing a race only to realize the finish line was just the very beginning. A little overwhelmed, I figured that the first thing I should do was decide which school I wanted to attend. And then what? Just show up, I supposed, in hopes that someone would tell me what to do when I got there. I sent in a response letter accepting my spot and was duly enrolled in the Class of 2003 at the Columbia University College of Physicians and Surgeons, affectionately referred to by the diminutive "P and S."

Despite the fact that both of my parents had completed the training process themselves, I didn't have any real sense of what medical school was going to be like. Both of them would dredge up some old stories when I asked, but these stories were more nostalgia pieces about the cafeteria food or the bike frame my dad somehow nailed into the concrete wall of his dorm room, rather than anything that I *really* wanted to know. And all pretense about academics and clinical experience aside, what I really wanted to know boiled down to nothing more than what a young child asks before embarking on her first summer at sleepaway camp: *What's it going to be like? What will we do every day? Will I have friends? If I decide that I don't like it, can I come home?*

It is strange how some decisions that seem small at the time gain tremendous significance in retrospect. When I started the application process, I knew only that I wanted badly to attend medical school in New York City, the city where I had grown up and where my family still lived. Beyond that, I had very little preference. By the end of the application process, I had narrowed down the decision to two medical schools in Manhattan, but it was a tough call deciding between the two. My parents, I think, would have preferred me to attend NYU, not just because my father had completed his Dermatology residency there but because they felt the neighborhood was safer than the one around Columbia, the medical campus of which was so far north that it was practically an annex of the Bronx. In the end, I ended up choosing Columbia for only the vaguest reasons—the students I met there during my interview seemed nice, and I thought I might fit in better there. *What if no one likes me? Who will I sit with during lunch? What if I drop my tray in the cafeteria and everyone laughs at me?*

The first evening of my medical school orientation, during a particularly steamy week in late August, there was a meet-and-greet barbecue on the roof of the dormitory where most of the first-year medical students were housed—that is to say, before we knew any better and all fled to superior accommodations. I was tired from my day of moving in and running between various administrative offices and almost decided to skip the event entirely, opting instead to head back downtown and rest at my parents' apartment, where at least I knew that the refrigerator was stocked and the air-conditioning worked. In the end, however, I decided that I should make at least *some* effort to be social and forced myself to trudge upstairs to the rooftop—where stored heat still rose from the tile at 8:00 p.m.—politely accepted a watered-down beer from one of several weathered-looking kegs rolled up for the occasion, and answered and asked the same five questions over and over and over again: *What's your name? Which room are you in? Where are you from originally? Where did you go to college? What was your major? Really? Wow. That's interesting. Wow.*

I rolled over to the next person to my left—this meet-and-greet was starting to resemble some kind of bizarre receiving line, and gamely asked my intro questions for the umpteenth time: "Hi! How's it going? What's your name?"

"Joe." He was medium height, with short-cropped sandy hair, blue eyes rimmed with smile lines so deep they never seemed to completely go away.

"Joe? Your name is *Joe*?" That day, I had already met a Mehul, an Olan, an Amit, a Sreedavi, a Tao, and a Kar-Fei. Never being very good with names, I was already envisioning weeks, if not *months*, of stealthily employed mnemonics, face-recognition flashcards, and embarrassing mispronunciations that would forever brand me not only as culturally insensitive but also kind of idiotic. And for the first time that evening, I said something completely spontaneous. "Thank *God* your name is *Joe*!"

His smile lines got deeper, his eyes twinkly. "Why, is that your name too?"

"No! *No*. Michelle. I'm Michelle."

I didn't know this back then, but I would eventually marry this man, who ten years later would be the father of my two beautiful boys and a sensitive and talented oculoplastic surgeon besides. But back then I didn't know any of what lay ahead. All I knew then was that he was yet another fresh face in the crowd, a medical student on his very first day of school, just like me.

Preclinical

My second year of medical school, the United States Army came out with a new print and TV ad campaign aimed at recruitment; the slogan (previously "Be All That You Can Be") was updated to "You Are An Army of One," emphasizing strength and individualism. *Come join us!* the ads seemed to implore. *Tap your full potential, and kick a little ass while you're at it!* One day before lecture, my classmate Bea and I were discussing these new ads and the fresh public image that the Army was eager to project.

"The Army has these new ads because people think being in the Army *sucks,*" Bea observed. "The general perception that people have is that the Army is all about pointless drills that break your spirit, being demoralized and harassed by higher ranking officers, getting no sleep, having no social life, never going out on dates, and spending the majority of your day crawling around in the mud. So I guess these new ads are supposed to change our minds."

"Yeah, good luck with that," I drawled, flipping through my lecture notes and fishing through my bag for a pen.

Bea paused. "But the thing is, all those things that people think about the Army...that's what *med school* is like. That's exactly my life *now.* Well, except for the crawling-around-in-the-mud part."

"Speak for yourself, Bea."

* * *

30

Army analogies aside, the fact of it is that the first two years of medical school are surprisingly like— and I don't necessarily mean this in a bad way—prison. At least in college, people had different majors, took different classes, traveled in separate circles. A med school class is more like a chain gang of 150 convicts locked together at the ankles for four years. Every single class, every exam, every lecture, every panel discussion, we attended together. Factor in the fact that all of us had at one time been premed, and right there you have a claustrophobic terrarium of type A personalities thriving and occasionally cannibalizing each other in our natural habitat.

But perhaps that's a little extreme.

Though essentially it came down to a coin toss, one of the reasons that I chose to attend Columbia was, as I mentioned earlier, because of the student body. The selection process for any medical school is rigorous, such that you can pretty much be assured that anyone who has made it far enough to be accepted is reasonably intelligent, with a high GPA and good MCAT scores. But a good medical student on paper is not always a good medical student to spend four years of your life with. In my premedical student cohort in college, I knew premeds who were so competitive that they would without reservation stab you in the back with the jagged ends of a broken Erlenmeyer flask if it meant advancing their own agendas. I knew premeds who seemed to have no outside interests other than studying for exams and, afterward, reliving said exams, question by question, line by line in excruciating and (need it be said) pointless detail. I knew premeds who ate their own nails, who seemed not to notice that articles of their clothing were on inside-out, who would examine a bottle of shampoo with a quizzical expression, either in the process of diagramming its molecular components or (worse yet) trying to figure out what exactly shampoo was used for. I did not want to go to school with those people.

Columbia, being a reasonably well-regarded medical school, has the luxury of choosing students who are not just good on paper. Many of them are interesting and funny and shockingly *normal* as well. I liked this, though I couldn't—*still* can't—figure out for the life of me how I managed to get admitted myself. Hanging out with medical students who were normal made *me* feel a little more normal myself for essentially signing away the next eight to ten years of my life as an indentured servant to the medical machine.

But no matter where you are, the fact of it is that medical school is a lot of mind-bendingly hard work in one of the most hierarchical environments outside of the armed forces. And then there is the studying and the studying, and after that, there's *more* studying. Have some free time? Why not study? It is like college finals week inflated to monstrous proportions, and instead of lasting a week, it lasts *years*. And perhaps the most pernicious consequence of all this is not the fatigue or the repetition or the sheer amount of brute memorization required, it's that studying all day every day forces you to be alone a lot.

So despite the fact that medical students are by

their very nature competitive, despite the fact that there is only so much room at the top of each class, we are all in some way grateful for our classmates. Because the only people who can understand what it's really like to be a medical student are people who are in medical school themselves.

* * *

It was the fall of my first year, and the hallway outside the anatomy lab was filled with half-naked med students.

In medical school, anatomy lab is a rite of passage in which, traditionally, preserved cadavers are dissected in an effort to teach the medical neophyte all she could want or need to know about the intricacies of the human body. Of course, the idea of the anatomy curriculum is a holdover from an earlier age—back before a more detailed understanding about physiology and pharmacology and genetics, all they *could* teach in medical school was what was visible to the naked eye. But despite its growing obsolescence as the focal point of any medical student's induction into the world of preclinical practice, it is still a respected and honored course, one that, at Columbia at least, started our first week of medical school and extended well into the spring, at which point the rising temperatures outdoors and open windows of the anatomy lab led the course to a swift and merciful conclusion. (No matter how dedicated to our studies, the presence of those first few flies flitting from this exposed femur to that desiccated eyeball brought what exactly we were doing—which was fishing around elbow-deep in the guts of dead people—starkly into relief.)

Due to the strong smell in the anatomy lab and the quasitoxic preservatives used to keep the cadavers if not exactly *fresh*, at least *intact*, we all changed into scrub suits before anatomy lab. Some people washed their scrubs every week, some didn't wash their scrubs at all, but no one eschewed a change of scrubs entirely. The anatomy lab smell was powerful and stomach turning, and despite all precautions, I still caught whiffs of it on my skin or in my hair sometimes even days after our lab sessions ended.

Outside the dissecting labs were banks of lockers lining the hallways where we kept our clothes and dissection kits, and due to the lack of a proper locker room, these hallways were where most of the medical students changed before class. Some of the more demure students (mostly women, a few shy men) found an empty amphitheater or fire escape to duck into before doffing their street clothes, but most of us at this point had lost all modesty and didn't think much of getting changed in front of our classmates. After all, we were standing outside a giant room in which thirty dead people were lying naked on metal tables under harsh fluorescent lighting. What was the embarrassment in seeing 150 half-clad live ones?

As I was changing into my jade green scrubs printed with the medical school logo (we had been told sternly and repeatedly by the dean of students herself that as first-year students we were *only* to wear *green* scrubs; *blue* scrubs, meanwhile, were to be worn only by *senior* students within the hospital building—the vigor with which she punctuated this edict only accentuating our sense of being lower-caste members, now distinguishable not only by experience but also by color), I saw Joe changing down the hall from me. We hadn't spoken much since we initially met at the rooftop barbecue a few months earlier. He was well muscled like an athlete and had, improbably, a large colorful tattoo on his left upper arm, which, even at this distance, I could identify as some sort of tropical bird, with a long tail feather fanning out up over his shoulder. It was the kind of tattoo you'd expect to see on a blue-collar tough guy, like an auto mechanic or a construction worker, and its incongruity in this setting intrigued me. As though sensing my analysis, Joe looked up from tying his scrub pants, and, flustered, I turned away, pretending to purge my dissecting kit of cadaveric flotsam before closing my locker and heading into the lab.

After class, after we had all changed back into street clothes and most of us had already stepped back out into the early dusk of mid-November, back to a night at the dorms where we would (of course) study, Joe approached me, a friendly smile on his face.

"You're from New York, right?" he asked without a prelude.

"Yeah," I said, trying to remember whether or not we'd had this conversation before. "I used to live downtown near NYU."

"Oh good." He actually looked relieved. "Do you know any toy stores in the city where I could buy presents for some kids I know?"

Kids? I thought. *What kids?* Your *kids?* Also, *There's apparently this thing called the Internet designed for just such store-finding tasks as this!* Thankfully, I said neither of these things. "Toy stores? Well, yeah. Sure I know where you could go."

After considering my options—FAO Schwarz was too touristy and expensive, some of the more boutique-type toy stores I knew didn't have a very large selection—I started telling Joe about the large Toys "R" Us below Times Square and explained to him how to get there by taking the A train down from our dorms in Washington Heights. "Or," and I paused, wondering why the hell I was saying this—he was a grown man after all and could certainly follow a set of directions and a subway map, "I could just *show* you. I'm headed toward there this weekend myself anyway."

This was a rather large lie. Herald Square, the neighborhood around this particular Toys "R" Us, was perhaps the patch of land I most despised in all of Manhattan—always noisy and gridlocked and teeming with harassed shoppers trampling one another to find the best deal on discounted irregular hosiery at Daffy's—but I had a very strong desire to have a conversation with this guy Joe outside of the confines of medical school, not standing in front of a bank of lockers while reeking of cadaver preservative.

"You are? Great! I just need to pick up some stuff there. I'm visiting some friends and their kids for Thanksgiving, and I want to bring presents." *Nice guy,* I thought to myself, making a mental list. *Good guest. Likes kids.* We made plans to meet up on

Saturday (I had originally planned to study for most of the day, but more out of habit than any particular urgency) and after some minimal friendly small talk, we parted ways for the evening. I considered walking away whistling, hands in pockets, but in the end figured that this was perhaps too theatrical a charade of nonchalance to disguise the fact that I was actually completely thrilled.

Was there dating in medical school? Yes, of course there was, how could there not be? Convenience aside—how else was the time-pinched student ever supposed to *meet* anyone?—dating within a medical school came along with an instant shorthand and understanding of the other person's obligations. Some couples formed quickly and insolubly, others were more casual, joining and separating and rejoining again as convenience or our exam schedule permitted. Many people in our class were in relationships with people outside of medicine, which they claimed was necessary for maintaining both their identity and sanity. But many others were part of medical couples, some with partners or spouses in other fields of medicine, sometimes several years apart in training. The advantages of this were clear as well. *You don't have to explain,* one partner could tell the other, either during a tough night on call or in the painful efforts of condensing the contents of an entire bookshelf into a modest-looking grayish pink organ the size of a cantaloupe. *I went to medical school too, and I know exactly what you're going through.*

Years later, a few weeks before Joe and I got married, one of our medical school classmates, Tim, offered as a wedding gift a snapshot of us from what Tim calls our "first date." The photo is from a class party the night after our first-semester finals in December, downtown at a seedy bar called McSorley's. In the picture, Joe and I are sitting together, leaning toward each other; my arm is around his shoulder, and we are both grinning like idiots. It's not a particularly flattering picture of either of us, but from looking at it you can tell that Joe and I like each other a lot, maybe even more than a lot, and are just happy to have an excuse to spend time together.

There are plenty of pictures from medical school that are unmistakably med-student photos—our graduating-class yearbook is full of them: Pictures of our classmates standing around stiffly in our freshly pressed short white lab coats. Gag pictures of people taking stethoscopes and listening to each other's heads with bemused expressions, or standing next to a mounted human skeleton, pretending to take a pulse and finding it sadly lacking. Stealthy hidden-camera–type pictures taken of our classmates asleep facedown on a microbiology textbook, or frowning over a patient's chart on the wards. There are plenty of photos of us looking like medical students. But I like this picture that Tim gave us because in it, we look like regular people.

It would be a nice story if this photo of us at McSorley's really *was* from our first date. But actually, there was no one there to take pictures of our *real* first date, which was spent wandering the aisles of Toys "R" Us in Herald Square, searching up and down the shelves for that perfect toy for a one-year-old boy in San Francisco named Armando, picking up and discarding a number of educational and intellectually stimulating options before deciding in the end, *screw it,* and buying him a big box full of plastic bugs instead.

* * *

The first two years of medical school, the preclinical years, are not very memorable, because honestly, so much of this time is spent in the insular pursuit of knowledge that sometimes days could go by, one after the other, all identical but for which page of the syllabus I happened to be turned to at the time. I'd once heard an analogy that stuck with me because it was so true: in high school, they feed you information with a spoon; in college, they feed you information with a bucket; and in medical school, they feed you information with a fire hose. And sometimes, around midterms, they feed you with a fire hose while administering a colonic. So really, can you blame me for not being able to remember much?

It is strange how a culture of learning so dependent on rote memorization yields so few experiential memories in and of itself. To paraphrase Sartre, Hell may well be other people, but at least with other people around, you can confirm that you are *indeed* in Hell—nod, laugh, commiserate, elbow each other in the side and shout, *Hot enough for ya?* And if you try hard enough and the right people are along for the ride, you can actually occasionally have some fun.

Like it or not, this is how doctors are made.

Four Short Plays About the Preclinical Years of Medical School

1. DERMATOMES

(SCENE: A medical school dorm room, October 30, 2000. JOE and MICHELLE are getting dressed for the big medical school Halloween party, held every year in the appropriately, though not intentionally, grim and somewhat haunted-appearing basement of the medical school dormitory. They have coordinating costumes and are going as "The Dermatomes," a graphic representation of the areas of skin on the human body supplied by a single spinal nerve. This costume, misguidedly perceived to be wildly humorous and innovative by its sadly nerdish creators, involves both parties donning full-length black unitards inscribed with puffy glitter paint in wavy horizontal lines and spinal cord levels. Having not planned ahead, JOE and MICHELLE have left the actual glitter painting for the last twenty minutes before the party, but as with most things in medical school, there is a lesson to be learned from this as well.)

JOE: These costumes are going to be awesome!

MICHELLE: Awesome!

JOE: *Awesome!*

MICHELLE: Wait, hold still a second, let me get this right. *(Laboriously, consulting Netter's* Atlas of Human Anatomy *for guidance, completes drawing one line across JOE'S nipple line, which she labels "T4")* There. One level down, only twenty-nine to go. Wait, twenty-*nine* more dermatomes, right? I don't think I paid enough attention in Anatomy.

JOE: Yeah, twenty-nine more. And then I have to do your costume. It's OK, we still have fifteen minutes left.

(One-and-a-half hours later.)

JOE: Oops, I think I smudged your T8 level.

MICHELLE: Dude, just hurry up! The party's going to be *over* by the time we finish! And I haven't even done your back or any of your lumbar or sacral levels yet. I don't think we have time. Or enough puffy paint.

JOE: But the bull's-eye over the ass is the key part! That's what makes the whole look!

MICHELLE: Forget it, man, no one's going to look at our *legs*! We're not going to have anywhere to wear these costumes if we take much longer! Just finish up my torso and let's just get downstairs before all the booze is gone.

JOE: *(Shaking empty glitter paint tube)* I think I'm out here. What next? Do you have one of those Wite-Out pens?

MICHELLE: Just forget it, it's good enough. Also, you failed to note what a fine job I did on your arms. Getting C6, C7, and C8 to line up in three dimensions wasn't easy.

JOE: I'm surprised you didn't use up all the paint just on my massive guns. *(Flexes)*

MICHELLE: Don't smear the paint, Mister Universe, you're not dry yet. Just finish T10 on me, will you? No one's going to look below my belly button, they'll get the gist of the costume.

JOE: It *is* an awesome costume.

MICHELLE: For sure. The Dermatomes! *To a med school Halloween party!* Classic! People are going to *love* this!

(Twenty minutes later, in the dimly lit basement. The DJ is playing Britney Spears, and a score of female medical students, all dressed as some iteration of "naughty schoolgirl," squeal and start dancing enthusiastically.)

MICHELLE: *(Walking up to SEJAL, another medical student, who is watching this scene with detached amusement)* Hey, Sejal, how's it going. Where's your costume?

SEJAL: Oh, I don't have one, I'm going to a real party after this, and I don't want to look stupid. *(Beat)* Hey, but look, *you're* wearing a costume! What are you supposed to be, a mime?

MICHELLE: What? No, not a *mime*. No! Joe and I are The Dermatomes. *Dermatomes*. See? *(Points to her chest, where, barely visible, is a faint paint line and the letters "T5")* Like in Anatomy class, get it?

SEJAL: Oh yeah. *(Smiles politely)* It's hard to see that writing in here. Because, you know, it's sort of dark.

MICHELLE: But we used *glitter paint*.

SEJAL: *(Edging away)* So...I'm going to get something to drink.

JOE: *(Wandering back from the refreshment table)* Got you a beer.

MICHELLE: Oh, thanks. You know, Sejal just thought I was dressed as a mime?

JOE: What? Please. Does a *mime* have spinal nerve levels written on his arms and chest? Does a *mime* consult an anatomy atlas to figure out how to dress? Really.

MICHELLE: I know, right? Sejal's crazy. Hey look, there's Andy and Jess. They're wearing matching costumes too.

(ANDY approaches, wearing a nylon jogging suit, a visor, and clutching a badminton racket. JESS, identically attired, is puttering forward gamely with a cloud of talcum powder rising from her dusted hair. They are "retired.")

ANDY: Hey, Joe and Michelle! What are you supposed to be? Cat burglars?

MICHELLE: *(Apoplectic)* We are dermatomes! *Dermatomes!* Aren't you supposed to be in *medical school*? Aren't you guys supposed to *know* this stuff? It took us two hours to draw these dermatomes on our clothing and I want people to *acknowledge* that these costumes are a freaking work of art!

(RYAN wanders by, wearing a bonnet, a pacifier, a diaper, and a short-cropped T-shirt reading MOMMY'S LITTLE SWEETHEART.)

RYAN : Joe, Michelle, what's up! Cool costumes!

MICHELLE : *Yes!* I mean...thank you!

RYAN : What are you, like, *Cirque du Soleil* or something?

2. HEART

(SCENE: Gross Pathology lab, medical school classroom. Insert "Gross! Pathology!" joke here. The class has been broken up into smaller groups of four or five students and has been given a mound of pathologic human hearts to catalog. Unfortunately, there is no instructor present, which means that any learning that may take place will be purely accidental. Additionally, there is also something vaguely unseemly about watching these medical students fumbling their way through the basics of medical science, knowing that in just two and a half years, these same people are going to be actual doctors, performing surgery and prescribing medications for your baby's ear infection. It's a little like watching a skinny adolescent Arnold Schwarzenegger starting to train using a pair of tiny, pink rubber-coated five-pound free weights. A necessary first step, but somehow embarrassing to witness.)

MICHELLE : *(Picking up a dripping heart from the tray)* So this heart...is really big. That's bad. Right? Bad.

AMRESH : *(Nodding)* Yeah. I say seriously bad.

MICHELLE : Hearts should not be this big. This patient has, like, problems. He has, uh, what's that word they said in lecture today? Cardio...megaly?

AMRESH: Yeah, and...um...dilatation and hypertrophy.

MICHELLE: Ooh, check out the professor here. Nice! *(Flipping through the heart, which has helpfully been bisected prior to arriving in the classroom)* His valves look fine, but what the hell do I know. Man, this heart is huge.

BOB: I think it's a cow heart. Do you think that's part of the weeding-out process? They stick a cow heart in the pile and you have to figure out which one it is? And if you don't pick up on it they kick you out of med school? *(Pause)* It's possible, is all I'm saying.

MICHELLE: Look at his...you know...what do you call these little things? *(Fingering the little slips of heart tissue anchoring the valves)*

AMRESH: Oh, those are...um...oh, I forget.

MICHELLE: They're called...uh...wait wait, I got it, they're...papillary muscles?

AMRESH: *(Excited)* Right! Yes! *(High-fives MICHELLE. Heart juice splashes off their gloved hands.)* Ew.

MICHELLE: Hey, you know when I was in high school, we had to do this fetal pig dissection? And there was this kid in my class who said that for fifty dollars, he would eat a piece of the pig heart, like, with the preservative and everything? And someone actually *gave* him fifty dollars, and he *did* it! True story!

(Silence.)

MICHELLE: Yes, well, anyway. *(Handling a different specimen)* Hey now, what the hell is all *this*?

AMRESH: What?

MICHELLE : *(Points to strange mass in the right atrium)* This squishy thing.

AMRESH : Oh, I don't know.

MICHELLE : This reminds me of taking Anatomy last year. Every time we found a structure that we didn't recognize, we would just say it was some tumor and move on.

AMRESH : When in doubt—*tumor*.

MICHELLE : Right on.

AMRESH : Shameful.

MICHELLE : Oh, like *you* know what it is.

AMRESH : I don't. But I bet it's bad.

MICHELLE : *All* these hearts look bad.

AMRESH : Which probably explains why all these people are dead. *(Picking up another heart, turning it over in his hands)* I'm not too sure what we're supposed to be looking at here.

MICHELLE : You know what, when you're a pathologist, this is just all you do all day long. It's like being in Gross Pathology lab every *day* for the *rest* of your *life*.

AMRESH : Well, that's another career to cross off my list, then.

3. Patterns of Inheritance

(SCENE: Medical school housing complex, MICHELLE'S apartment, evening. Her parents have dropped by for a visit. These visits are enjoyed by all—MICHELLE loves it anytime someone drops by her Den of Sweat and Toil, as it grants necessary respite from the ceaseless grind of medical school study, and besides, her

parents often bring food and mail and proof that the outside world does, indeed, exist. Her mother and father, she presumes, enjoy these visits as well—aside from a chance to see their firstborn in a most satisfying state of overwrought academia, it allows them to relive their own medical school memories, by this point sepia-toned and overly romanticized.)

MOM: *(Inspecting dusty plants languishing on the windowsill, which MICHELLE purchased during a fit of optimism that she might ever remember to water any plants in her care)* This one's getting all yellow for some reason.

DAD: *(Heartily, staring out the window at the resplendent view of the George Washington Bridge and the great state of New Jersey)* Wow! What a view! When *I* was in med school, we didn't have housing as nice as *this*! We lived in a cinder block dorm and I used to sneak into the Jewish students' dorms because they had better food!

MOM: You have to water it. Are you watering it?

MICHELLE: I *know* you have to water plants, Ma. I *did* water it.

MICHELLE'S INNER MONOLOGUE: Once.

DAD: I'll bet you have the best view in the building!

MICHELLE: Yeah, we're pretty high up. Remember when there were those brownouts in this neighborhood last summer because too many people were using their air conditioners? I had to walk down thirty-one flights to get to class. Which was still better than having to walk thirty-one flights back *up* to get home.

MOM: You have to pick off the dead leaves. See, like this. *(Pick, pick, pick)*

MICHELLE'S INNER MONOLOGUE: There's a giant hairball right on the rug there. I forgot to vacuum the floor again. My parents are going to think I just lie here, slowly moldering in a pile of my own excreta as, slowly, my Pharmacology syllabus threatens to consume me. Why didn't I vacuum?

MICHELLE: *(Kicking hairball behind a chair)* Yeah. Pick off the dead leaves. Got it.

DAD: Look, you can see the skyline! This view is *great*! Oh, how is Joe, by the way?

(MICHELLE has just recently introduced Joe to her parents, despite great trepidation leading up to this event, because no amount of dim lighting can disguise the fact that JOE is A White Man and therefore instantly suspect in the eyes of her zeroth generation Chinese parents. However, being clean cut and having a master's in Chemistry from UC Berkeley apparently counts as being Chinese enough, and so Joe has been accepted into the fold with a minimum of parental protest.)

MICHELLE'S INNER MONOLOGUE: Oh man, *The Guide to Getting It On* on my desk right between my stapler and Scotch tape dispenser. I can't believe I didn't move the sex book before my parents came over. Please, please, don't look over now...

MICHELLE: *(Deftly moving a pile of index cards to cover the offending title)* Hey, look over here! I got a new textbook for my Physical Diagnosis class! You know, where we learn how to examine patients? See how it has all these cool pictures of the different parts of the physical exam! *(Flips book open randomly, landing on the page with large diagrams of the pelvic exam. Quickly slams book shut.)*

DAD : *(Picking up the proffered textbook, fingering its leatherette spine)* Hmm. Bates' Guide to Physical Examination and History Taking. We used this too. When *we* were in med school. *(Smiling at the recollection)* I still remember when your mom came over to my dorm room that first time. She said she needed to borrow my notes from class. Of course, I *knew* that was an excuse, but I played along, you know.

MOM : You know what you might need? Plant food!

4. EXAMS

(SCENE: The week before the big Infectious Disease midterm, which, if we are to believe the hype, is the most important exam ever in the history of the universe, quite possibly also in parallel universes. DR. PRINCE, a medical instructor of the old school, neither suffers fools nor hesitates to make this point. At this moment she is attempting to revive the flagging spirits of the second-year students by giving them something of a pep talk, though in her inimitable way, her pep talk only manages to make everyone feel more suicidal.)

DR. PRINCE : Look, you guys are making *way* too

much of this. This exam is going to be easy! Easy easy easy! *If you study. (Suddenly menacing)* Are you studying?

CLASS: *(Rendered mute with fatigue)*

DR. PRINCE: Look, the test, I wrote it. It's a fair test. Any microbiologist would do just fine on the test.

CLASS: *(An uneasy rustling, as the gathered crowd in the lecture hall come to realize that, with rare exception, none of them are microbiologists)*

DR. PRINCE: Like look, Dr. Lowy here. *(She points to DR. LOWY sitting in the front row, bespectacled faculty expert on streptococcus and closest available comic foil.)* Dr. Lowy would do fine on this exam. *(Pause)* He wouldn't get a perfect score. But he would pass it. Probably.

CLASS: *(Loud weeping)*

(Later that evening, MICHELLE and JOE are having a study session at JOE'S apartment. Beside them are two empty liquid mush bowls, because when you are a medical student during exam season, it doesn't matter what you eat or how it tastes, so long as the foodstuff can be made in a single giant pot at the beginning of the week in sufficient volume to last you until Friday, or until you've eaten it so many days in a row that even the sight of it sends you into a cold sweat. This week's iteration of feed is mushroom-barley soup.)

MICHELLE: So maybe we should talk over some of these old exam questions. I hear they reuse the multiple-choice questions a lot.

JOE: The answer is C!

MICHELLE: We didn't start yet.

JOE: Oh. I change my answer to B then.

MICHELLE: OK, first question. The cell attachment proteins on viruses of the *Paramyxoviridae* family—

JOE: Tuberculosis.

MICHELLE: I didn't even get to the question yet. Anyway, that's wrong.

JOE: Doesn't matter. Tuberculosis is the answer to everything.

(JOE'S roommate DAVE enters, returning from the library.)

DAVE: Oh, are you guys going over exam questions? I've just been reading all day, I need to do questions. Can I study with you guys?

MICHELLE: Only if you don't actually care about passing the exam.

(Two days later, after the exam, JOE and MICHELLE are out celebrating their one-year anniversary. In actuality, their anniversary was a few days before, but the medical school exam schedule did not care, and so they are celebrating belatedly. Tonight they are at Dallas BBQ, which, not surprisingly, is a barbecue restaurant universally beloved by the student body for its enthusiastic and unabashed embrace of all things meat.)

MICHELLE: I would have gotten ribs, since we're cel-

51

ebrating, but I think that eating ribs in public makes me look ridiculous.

JOE: Yeah, brisket is the way to go.

MICHELLE: I feel like I should get a beer or something, but I swear if I drink anything with alcohol in it, I will just fall asleep immediately. I can barely even sit up now.

JOE: I hear you. Man, I have so much laundry to do. I've been waiting until after this exam, but now I'm down to my last pair of underwear.

MICHELLE: Just wear it inside-out tomorrow.

JOE: Huh?

MICHELLE: Nothing. Oh hey, look at the size of that guy's soda! Is that the "Texas-sized" drink?

JOE: Huh? *(Looks)* I suppose so.

MICHELLE: Oh man, I'm getting a Texas-sized Diet Coke. I am so excited! Not only will I get a Texas-sized caffeine bolus, I'll also get to drink out of a giant goblet like in Medieval Times.

JOE: I'm glad you're so excited. So, what do you want to do after this? We could go out to celebrate. I think the class is having a party downtown at that place...

MICHELLE: Oh, at that bar? Meh. I'm sick of hanging out with other medical students. Anyway, everyone's just going to be talking about the test, and I don't think I want to hear it right now. Besides, I think I have to get up early to study tomorrow for Pharmacology. I've been so busy studying for that other exam, I haven't looked at my Pharm notes at all.

JOE: Well, what *do* you want to do then?

MICHELLE: Honestly? After we eat? Let's just go home and sleep.

JOE: *(Relieved)* Really? Thank god. That's what I want to do too.

MICHELLE: Sweet sweet sleep, the best date night of all.

JOE: Happy anniversary, honey. I love you.

MICHELLE: Love you too.

* * *

And so the first two years of my medical training passed by in a hazy blur, and where we could, most of us tried to have some fun and retain a sense of humor—not easy in those two years, when it felt as though you were moving through the gears of a machine determined to crush you into compact, equally sized stackable blocks of facts and numbers.

While the divisions in medical school are fairly well demarcated—the first two years are almost entirely preclinical, spent not in the hospital with patients but in the classroom with books—over the years the faculty and administration developed the sense that they had to give the first- and second-year med students a sense of what they were studying *for*, lest they lose their way and meander toward a career in medical consulting or (worse yet) business school. So every once in a while, preclinical students are offered a taste of the actual practice of medicine, either shadowing a doctor on the wards, spending a night on the labor and delivery floor, or being lectured to by one of the clinical staff on some aspect of patient care. Occasionally, there would be a particular lecture where a patient was brought in and bandied about like some sort of exotic zoo creature (at which point all of us in the assembled audience would fall over ourselves trying to best each other with The Most Sensitive Question: "So, what did it *feel like* when you were diagnosed with Huntington's disease?"), but on the whole, the first two years of medical school were an insular time. Sometimes it was even hard to *remember* why we are doing it all—at points it got to feeling like the reason we were studying about renal pathophysiology was not so much to be able to help our future patients with renal disease, but rather to help *ourselves* get a good grade on the renal pathophysiology final exam. It was easy to lose sight of the big picture.

There is an essential change in thinking for medical students transitioning from the second to third year of medical school. You go from a program of purely self-directed activity where you are working for yourself, *by* yourself, to a program wherein every moment of every day involves working in a team, wholly for the benefit of strangers who have for one reason or another entrusted themselves to your care. Basically, we had to pull out our med school applications, dust off the essays that we had written, and try to remember why we had come here in the first place. We had to relearn altruism.

Most of us were ready for this, had been waiting for the chance to crawl out from under the deadfall of textbooks and finally, *finally* start to learn what we had come to med school to do. Occasionally this transition is a little difficult to negotiate, but eventually it becomes second nature, to the point that we eventually no longer question placing a patient's needs before our own. Our patients are sick, relatively powerless in the shadow of the medical machine, and they need us to help them. And over time we do so almost instinctively, without thinking, like parents helping a child put on a winter coat, or leading an aged relative carefully down a set of stairs.

So there we were, young and idealistic and almost hyperactive with the notion of finally being set free, like a gang of kids who, after a long flight with two layovers and a three-hour taxi into the gate, are finally released to run free on the tarmac. We had all the good intentions and energy in the world. We knew *everything*. We could do *anything*. And even if there were situations beyond our ability, just a little bit outside our experience or reach, well, at least we were *there*, and we *cared*. (Perhaps a clenched jaw and a shake of the fist was called for at this last bit. Also, background music. There would always be background music.)

Not until the first time we had to set foot in the hospital did we realize this: *we had absolutely no idea what we were supposed to be doing.*

3 . CLINICAL PRACTICE

Welcome to the Monkey House

MY THIRD YEAR OF MEDICAL SCHOOL begins on the first of July. As opposed to the traditional Gregorian calendar, in which the year begins in January, the academic year in medicine begins in July, and as of today, I have been promoted from second-year medical student lost in the stacks at the library to third-year medical student, fresh scrubbed and shiny on the wards. *The wards.* Even just *saying* it makes me feel authentic. I am on Psychiatry, the first of ten five-week rotations designed to give us exposure to the full range of medical specialties. My first patient is an eighteen-year-old man who has just had his first psychotic break.

"What am I supposed to *do?*" I ask my resident, who seems inordinately occupied with some illegible progress note he is scribbling. I don't yet know this, but this will be the first of roughly 300 billion times I will ask that question this year.

"I don't know. It's your first day, so you can do whatever you want. Just go talk to him. Take a history." I am getting a definite *get lost* vibe from this resident, who is new here and trying to learn the ropes himself.

"But..." I want to ask him how I am supposed to take a history, but it seems like that might fall into the invisible category of "stupid questions." (Invisible because there aren't *supposed* to be any stupid questions except for those left unasked, but we all know that really, there *are* questions that are stupid, occasionally even *very* stupid. Like the time that, after an exhaustive hour-long lecture about human papillomavirus [HPV], one of my classmates raised her hands and asked with alacrity, "So...what *is* HPV anyway?"). I had taken medical histories before (How long have you had that cough?—that sort of thing) and I had even taken a few psych histories on fake patients—actors hired by the Psych Department to feign insanity so that we might hone our lines of questioning before being foisted upon the waiting masses. But I had never in my life taken a history from an actual psych patient.

So instead of asking my resident (who seems like he doesn't like me very much) the question I *really* want to ask, I ask him where I should conduct my interview. He points me toward an empty conference room and says, "I think you should be OK in there with the door closed, but let one of the nurses know you're going in there with him." I'm not sure if this last piece of advice is for my safety or for the patient's.

Andrew Hicks is not exactly overweight, but he walks laboriously, as though he has sandbags tied to every limb. After shuffling into the conference room, he sits perfectly still in the hard-backed chair and stares fixedly at me with absolutely no expression at all. Just sits there and stares. And *stares*. I remember from my Psych course second year that schizophrenics often display "flat affect" and "psychomotor retardation," which are just fancy words for what Andrew is doing, but overall, the effect is...well, it's pretty creepy.

"Well then," I say with what is probably an excess of volume and good cheer to make up for the vacuum in front of me. "My name is Michelle Au. I'm one of the medical students working here this month. If it's OK with you, I was wondering if we could talk a little about why you came into..." And here I pause briefly, my mind racing. What do I call this place? *The psych ward?* Is that pejorative? Will that offend him in some way? Out of nowhere, the phrase "nuthouse" pops into my head, and it capers irresistibly on the tip of my tongue. *Nuthouse, nuthouse, nuthouse.* "...the HOSPITAL," I say a little too loudly, to drown out this Greek chorus in my head. "Can you tell me why you came into the *hospital* last night?"

Andrew is apparently not offended. In a flat, low voice, with almost no inflection, he starts to tell me a long, complicated story, one which involves the Rosicrucian Order, the New York subway system, and the voice of God speaking to him from the intercom early yesterday morning. I interrupt a few times to get the progression of his symptoms straight, but after a while, I fall silent. "And that's how I know that I'm the son of God," Andrew finishes flatly, maybe twenty minutes later. I'm not really sure what to say to that last bit, so I just nod and repeat what he said.

He looks at me, his eyes dull behind his smeared glasses, his whole body unnaturally still, only his lips moving. "So, what do you think?"

"What do I think?" I'm not sure what he's getting at.

"Do you think I'm crazy?" And for the first time since we've started talking, I can tell what he's feeling. I can tell that he's afraid of what the answer will be.

I consider this question for what feels like a long time. What can you really say to a patient who asks you that? Especially after hearing him tell you the story he has, about sitting on the downtown A train and seeing hieroglyphics flashing overhead spelling out his name? About strangers on the street plotting to kill him, because they can see the power that he wields and are jealous of his "third eye"? I mean, really, what am I *supposed* to say?

"I think...that I'm glad that you're here with us, so that we can help you feel better." It's a glib answer, almost smarmy to my ear, and I can't tell quite how Andrew receives it. But he nods slowly, and after we decide to meet to talk further tomorrow, he lumbers awkwardly out of the room.

Exiting the room and walking into the glass-enclosed workstation, I see the head nurse sitting at a table on her lunch break. She eyes me, overearnest with my notepad, blindingly clean white coat (I would soon come to realize that no one else on the psych ward wore white coats, not even the attending physicians), a stethoscope dangling around my neck. She's older, in her sixties, and jaded like most senior nurses almost always become, having seen too much, done too much, and suffered through too many third-year medical students to count. She's probably thinking of a good many things she could say to me at this moment, her with her decades of experience and me still reeking of innocence and preservative from the anatomy lab. But all she tells me now, before spooning a bit of yogurt into her mouth, is this: "You shouldn't wear that stethoscope around your neck."

"Oh, really?" I look down at it, the black tubing draped on either side of my lapel. Was there a protocol or directionality to the thing that I wasn't aware of? Should I have the earpieces on the right instead of the left? "Why?"

Wordlessly, she stands up behind me, grabs both ends of my stethoscope, pulls it back so that the tubing is wrapped around my neck, and simulates twisting it tight, like a garrote. Jerking her head to indicate the patients on the other side of the glass, she says, "*That's* why."

* * *

It is now later in the day on the inpatient psych ward, and I am watching a patient go—and I believe this is the proper medical terminology—*totally apeshit.*

60

I'm not sure exactly what happened. He was standing in the hallway. One of the residents was talking to him. It looked like a pleasant exchange at first. The resident, a small, soft-spoken Asian man, was telling the patient something or other, smiling and gesturing comfortingly. The patient initially nodded, but suddenly the tide turned and his face turned an angry shade of plum, his craggy features knotting into something more sinister. Sensing danger, the resident started to back away. The patient, further enraged, picked up a nearby garbage can and hurled it full force at the resident, narrowly missing his head. The metallic clatter on linoleum was very loud, causing nurses at the station to jump and patients in the dayroom to look up from the TV, with the exception of one patient who never appeared to react to anything. And here we are now.

Overhead, I hear some hidden loudspeaker broadcasting, *"Psychiatric Emergency, all staff, Psychiatric Emergency,"* followed by the location of our ward. The personnel on our ward have all appeared, surging out from unseen corners and back rooms, followed by much of the security and support staff from the numerous other wards and offices in the building. Several burly security guards stand against the wall. This, I learn later, is called a *show of force*, a physical manifestation of the sheer manpower of the medical facility, in hopes that the patient will stand down peacefully, realizing that any efforts to try to fight his way out through the fifty or sixty people around him would be futile. I believe that law enforcement uses a similar method to subdue criminals, and that it works much of the time. A sane person would surely realize the uselessness of putting up a fight under such circumstances. But we are on an inpatient psychiatric ward. This guy is *crazy*.

True to form, the patient continues to rail and scream, throwing blind punches and gibbering incomprehensibly. The director of the ward, an impeccably dressed middle-aged attending of the gold-rimmed glasses, salt-and-pepper variety, approaches. I am cowering behind several larger staff members, but this attending actually walks up to the patient, like some sort of hostage negotiator in a movie. "You don't want to do this," he says quietly. He says something else softly that I can't hear, but I can see that he is gesturing toward the throng, appealing to the patient's sense of reason that it would be in his best interest to stand down, return to his room, maybe take a shot of what the staff call Vitamin H, their pet name for the powerful antipsychotic Haldol.

The patient is having none of it. "I'm not afraid of you!" he screams to the crowd in general. "Bring it on!" He throws another punch into the air, and suddenly, without warning, I see what appears to be a mattress running across the room. Actually, when I take a closer look, I see that it is actually three staff members holding up a twin mattress vertically, but even then, the effect is no less bizarre. The mattress has six legs and 500 pounds behind it, and in a matter of seconds, before the patient can react, it has pinned him up against the windows of the dayroom, where a number of other patients stand, goggle eyed.

Another nurse appears, a syringe is magically produced, and a swift intramuscular injection is administered amid muffled protest. The patient is moved swiftly to a protected isolation room, where he continues to scream hoarsely, infuriated at this latest subterfuge, until the screams get gradually groggier and groggier, and he eventually falls into a drugged doze. Two nurses and a security guard go in to check on him, and I can see from the door that the patient is snoring, lips flapping.

The crowd has since dispersed. My resident is already on his way to the next task but stops briefly to share with me a little pantomime, holding an invisible tube up to his mouth, taking aim, and then blowing sharply through it. When I look puzzled, he elaborates. "Haldol blow dart!" he says with a wink, and then, wisdom dispensed, he's on his way again. The patients are milling through the hallways as though nothing has happened. The nurses are in the back, busy dealing with stacks of patient charts. The director of the ward, the one who attempted negotiation with the patient, is by the nursing station, smiling as he rehashes the incident with another young attending. "He pretty much went crazy," I hear him say at one point, and they both laugh ruefully. *Are psychiatrists even allowed to refer to people as "crazy"?* I wonder. *After all that training and learning all those big psychiatric terms, the best they can come up with at this moment is "crazy"? That's like Einstein referring to light as "really fast."* Another patient walks by me, gangly and loose limbed, bobbing his head back and forth with each step like a chicken, making little *rrrhm rrrhm rrrhm* noises under his breath, as though revving a motor with each step.

This is my first day on the wards.

* * *

It is so early in my training and my experience is so limited that my most common impulse is to feel sorry for my patients, not only because they're sick and in the hospital, but because they have to be subjected to my fumbling and inexperienced ministrations in the name of medical education. Some patients *do* mind, and make their preferences clear, ranking medical students just under the janitorial staff and the lady who brings in their lunch trays, dismissing us with an indifferent wave of the hand or a stony glare that conveys just how useless to them we really are.

But on the whole, most patients do not mind our presence, and in fact *enjoy* having medical students around to talk to, to joke around with, to ask questions that the more senior doctors don't have time to answer. We are not yet as jaded as the nurses, are not as busy as the residents, and are nowhere near as unapproachable as the attendings. We have an easier time translating medical terms into plain language, because the chances are we recently had to surreptitiously look up those very terms ourselves. With one foot in each world, we are the perfect conduit between the edifice of medicine and the patient. And for the most part, the patients are happy to have us. During my first few months on the wards, I have had a grandmotherly patient invite me over for dinner, another invite me to her son's wedding, and yet another advise me earnestly about my plans for the future. (One in particular repeatedly asks me when I'm "going back to China," my frequent reminders that I was actually born in New York doing nothing to dissuade her from the notion that I need to "return to help my people.")

Sometimes, the patients are even a little *too* considerate. Early one morning, I am on the general medicine wards, rounding on one patient who just recently had a stroke resulting in some residual hemiparesis—that is, weakness and numbness on one side of his body. "Mr. Anderson," I start cheerily, though I don't know how cheerful *I'd* feel as the patient being shaken awake for a little 6:00 a.m. chat, "how are you feeling this morning?"

Mr. Anderson, shrugging diffidently, says only, "Mmm."

I continue, "Are you still feeling numb on your left side?"

He shrugs again, nods, and repeats, "Mmm."

Reaching down with the handle of my reflex hammer, I run the point lightly down Mr. Anderson's right shin and then his left. "Does this touch feel the same on both sides?"

He: "Mmm."

"Is that a yes or a no? Does it feel the same on both sides?"

"Mmm."

I reach down and grab each of Mr. Anderson's hands. "How about this? Does *this* feel the same? Or do you feel it more on one side?"

He shrugs, making a so-so gesture. "Mmm."

"Mr. Anderson, are you having problems speaking today?"

Averting his face, he only grunts again.

Starting to become concerned, I remind him, "You were speaking fine yesterday. Remember, we had that whole conversation about fishing? Is something wrong?" Again, he just shrugs and turns his head away from me. What is going on? Could he have had another stroke overnight? Is this an emergency? Should I call someone? Someone like a *real* doctor?

"Mr. Anderson"—my voice rising in volume seemingly out of my control—"what's the matter? Is it that you don't want to talk or that you *can't* talk?" More silence. "I need you to just say yes or no. Can you talk this morning? Open your mouth for me. Say 'Yes' or 'No.' " He keeps his head turned away, flicks his eyes back to mine, then presses his lips together even tighter.

What the hell is going on here? "Please tell me what's the matter. Why won't you talk to me? If you can, please try."

There is a long pause, then Mr. Anderson relents, whispers something through pursed lips.

Relieved that it seems that he can at least vocalize *something*, I ask, "What was that? I can't hear you. Could you say that again?"

Mr. Anderson, embarrassed, opens his mouth as little as possible and says very softly, "I haven't brushed my teeth yet this morning."

* * *

I am now on my Obstetrics and Gynecology rotation, sitting with an attending on teaching rounds, though it has rapidly become clear that, despite what anyone calls them, teaching is not necessarily the focus of these proceedings. Like a family of trained circus tigers, we as students are on display, participating in the great right of medical education known colloquially as "pimping."

Pimping, in essence, is a public trial in front of your peers. It involves being singled out by a senior, usually an attending, in front of some assembly, be it in a teaching conference, on rounds, or (most humiliatingly) at the patient's bedside, and being publicly interrogated on your medical knowledge. *Dr. Au, please give us eight causes of metabolic acidosis with an anion gap. In alphabetical order, please.* Depending on the mood of the attending, occasionally the question will go down the line from most-junior to most-senior member of the scrum, until finally, sometimes piecemeal, the desired answer is produced. If you are pimped and miss, your only recourse at this public humiliation is to blush, look down, furiously start consulting the index cards in your pocket, and hope that the correct answer, when provided—either by a more senior member of the squadron or perhaps another student better prepared than you—is not too humiliatingly easy.

The best kind of pimping involves a Socratic give-and-take between teacher and student, wherein the teacher probes the student to determine the limits of his understanding of the subject matter at hand (genetics, anatomy, miscellaneous Bible trivia) and, upon determining these limits, spurs an impromptu lecture on this that or the other thing, such that every member of the assembled audience will walk away awed and edified. However, at its worst, pimping involves the teacher asking rapid-fire questions he knows the student most likely cannot answer, and then gloating insufferably when the student fails to come through.

"Med students," one of the high-risk OB attendings now intones grandly, making sure that everyone in the room can hear him, "what amino-acid substitution is responsible for the mutation seen in sickle cell anemia?" He leans back grinning in his seat, professorial responsibilities presumably satisfied for the day. The other students and I look at each other, trying to figure out which one of us should field this one.

Finally I answer, the amino-acid substitution bubbling out of some unseen well of knowledge that I can access only involuntarily. "Glu to val," I blurt reflexively, like someone with a verbal tic. I cannot remember my PIN number for the ATM, barely can recall my own birthday, but two years of med school has given me the ability to recite medical factoids like Dustin Hoffman in *Rain Man*.

Instead of looking pleased, the attending glowers, and I realize then that he had been hoping for me to get the answer wrong. All signs are indicating that his pimping style is more of the "posit and gloat" variety. He frowns for a moment, and then counters, "Well, but what's the *codon* substitution?" asking not for the names of the amino acids, but rather the trinucleotide sequence of which it is composed. It is a question that may have some practical application in a molecular biology lab, but in this setting, with respect to bedside medicine, the information is not only arcane, it is essentially unimportant.

Springing out of the depths of this same dark repository of useless trivia, I want to say "GAG to GTG." I don't even know what this *means,* not quite sure what those letters stand for—what the hell is GAG to GTG?—but I can parrot the sequence back, for what it's worth. However, silently measuring my attending with my eyes, I can think of the better answer in this specific situation.

"I don't know."

As though I have just handed him a prize, the attending beams, gives a sharp bark of laughter, and looks around the room, as though to assess whether or not everybody heard my surrender. "You don't *know?* Well, you *should.* Why don't you do some reading about sickle cell tonight and give me a five-minute presentation tomorrow morning?" He adds in a tone that I presume is striving for magnanimous, "No PowerPoint slides necessary; handouts for the group will be fine."

Unable to help myself, I ask, "So...what *is* the codon substitution in sickle cell?" I arrange my face into what I think of as The Perfect Medical Student face, all at once sweet, hopeful, receptive, and reverent of authority. What I really want to know, though, is whether my attending is pimping me with questions he cannot answer himself.

There is a pause. "I have a scheduled C-section," he responds smoothly, looking at his watch, and without another word walks briskly out of the room.

Not speaking, I exchange glances with my fellow medical students, and when the moment seems right, we excuse ourselves from the room, exit into the hallway, and start laughing, one of us mimicking the attending's lightning-quick escape from any further "teaching."

This is how the third year of medical school has been so far, bouncing back and forth from the serious to the ridiculous, from the adult to the juvenile. There are moments of wonder and awe of course— my first day in the operating room, my first cardiopulmonary arrest on the wards, the first baby I saw born on Labor and Delivery. Each experience rendered me stunned and reverent for hours afterward. But what no one prepared us for was how *silly* life in the hospital can seem at times. The other night, as we were watching one of the women on the Labor and Delivery floor receive an epidural, the anesthesiologist told his patient casually before injecting the local anesthesia, "OK, you're going to feel a little prick in your backside," and it's all we could do not to start giggling right there.

Do I need to add at this point that we are of questionable maturity?

And that's the thing about medical students. Most of us *aren't* very old. We've all had our run-ins with patients who remark about how *young* doctors look these days, the more curmudgeonly among them asking us flatly in the middle of taking a history, "How old are you anyway? Twelve? Thirteen?" But the fact of it is that we *are* young. Those of us who went straight through to medical school—that is to say,

70

graduated from college and started medical school the following fall without taking any time off—were twenty-two years old at the start of our first year. I was actually even a little younger than most, the combination of skipping a grade and having a late-summer birthday meaning that I had turned twenty-one just a few weeks before I started medical school. Factor in the cloistered world of academics in which most medical students have been sequestered for at least the better part of a decade, along with (and I believe this is safe to presume) a predilection for bookishness, and the person whom you have entrusted with the task of your pelvic exam may not be quite as mature as you would hope.

Fortunately for us and sometimes unfortunately for our patients, medical students and residents do a lot of growing up on the job. The nature of medical training is such that the trainee is gradually, in an incremental fashion, put in a series of situations just one step beyond his or her level of comfort or expertise.

How does one bridge that gap from medical student to doctor? How does one *become* ready? I can only assume that one day, when the situation presents itself, I will have accumulated enough experience, have practiced enough, that stepping into the fray will feel natural and expected. But until then, I feel safe here, at the edge of the pool with my fellow medical students, all of us dipping our toes or one errant limb into the water but none of us quite daring to jump in.

We will all dive in eventually. And sometimes, we will be pushed.

Unforeseen Circumstances

It's 8:45 a.m. on a Tuesday morning, and I am in the OR watching some kid get circumcised.

Being the medical neophyte that I still am, watching a circumcision is still gruesome and fascinating in equal measure, but nowhere near as exciting as yesterday, when the senior Urology resident let me *do the actual circumcising* on a two-year-old patient with phimosis, a condition in which the foreskin becomes adherent to the head of the penis and can no longer be retracted.

"Here," he said offhandedly, giving me the scalpel and indicating where above the surgical clamp I should cut the foreskin. "Cut. All the way across."

It was my first time holding a scalpel, and I fingered its cool ridged handle, its surprising weight in my hand. "Really?" Not that I didn't want to get involved, but I just wanted to make sure that I'd, you know, *heard correctly*. The act of circumcision seemed simple enough, but of course, not being either a surgeon or a mohel, I'd never done this before. One slip, and twelve years later, I might have a very angry teenage boy show up on my doorstep.

"Sure," said the senior resident, bored already. Aside from the actual hassle of booking the OR time and putting the child under general anesthesia, the circumcision itself is a minuscule procedure for the surgeons, barely worth mentioning except in diminutives. "Just a circ," they say. Or is it *cirque*?

So I took the scalpel and cut, marveling at the smooth way the scalpel slid through the tissue, and the springy resistance the foreskin put up before being stripped away forever. In the end, the senior resident even let me put in a few stitches, hairlike filaments that held the foreshortened skin in place behind the shiny exposed glans, making it look under the bandage as though the kid's penis had sprouted whiskers.

But this morning, the attending himself is doing the circumcision, and Bob and I, the two medical students rotating through the Pediatric Urology service, are relegated to spectator status. Dr. Harris is one of the more senior urologists, gruff and of the old school, and I try to make myself small, hoping he won't even notice I'm there. Last week, when I was scrubbed in on a case with him, I forgot that I was sterile and absentmindedly reached up with a gloved hand to push up my glasses. The look of incredulous rage he shot me in that moment was enough to make me wonder if I had just ended my medical career right there and then.

The circ is progressing apace when, without warning, one of the nurses bursts in from outside, and I mean *bursts* in, as opposed to entering soundlessly and unobtrusively as we all try to (with the exception of the attending surgeons, who *always* burst in), and tells us, "Someone just crashed a plane into one of the Twin Towers."

What we all think instantly is that a small, one-engine plane, a tiny Cessna maybe, which had somehow gotten lost, spiraled out of control and clipped a wing on the edge of the building. "Cancel my reservation at Windows on the World!" Dr. Harris jokes bluffly, and a few people chuff or make the facsimile of laughter, perhaps to appease him. I don't say anything, but look at my classmate Bob, standing to my right, and make my eyes wide, in an *I-can't-believe-he-just-said-that* expression—eyes and brow being the only way one can silently and motionlessly communicate from behind a surgical mask. I figure that even if it *was* just a tiny little plane, there had to have been at least *some* damage, and at least one or two people must have gotten hurt.

The circumcision continues.

The same nurse now bursts in again, louder this time, and before she's even fully through the swinging double doors, she screams, "Someone just flew a plane into the other Tower! It's on fire!" And still, even then, I think that it must be some mistake. Some air traffic mishap maybe, or an obscuring cloud of smog, even though I know as much as anyone else who walked to work that the day outside is brilliantly sunny and clear, the epitome of Indian summer. It never crosses my mind at this point that it isn't an accident.

The nurse is now giving us updates from the live newscasts she has been watching out in the anesthesia conference room. They were huge passenger planes. They had flown directly into the Towers. The top floors are burning. People are trapped. We're wide-eyed, digesting this information, when another nurse enters the room, looking shaken. "Another plane just crashed into the Pentagon."

"Jesus Christ," Dr. Harris mutters. And then the room falls completely silent but for the steady beep of the anesthesia monitors, each of us absorbing the news.

Frantically, I think, *I have to call my family.* One of the nurses in the room is clearly thinking the same thing and starts dialing from the phone in the room. The volume on the handset is turned up high, and we can all hear the tinny beep of the busy signal.

Somehow we finish the case, the kid is bandaged and awakened, and together the team wheels him to Recovery. After talking with the parents and making sure that our patient is comfortable, one of the residents takes me and Bob to the tenth floor, and we walk over to the sky bridge up there, a long tube of metal and glass that connects the old hospital building to the new. It is here that we can finally get a view of what's going on in Lower Manhattan, more than two hundred blocks away.

This is the last time I will ever see the Twin Towers.

Even up in Washington Heights we can see them, like two giant smokestacks, steaming, choking black plumes billowing to one side, obscuring the tops of the buildings. From this distance, they look like lit cigarettes, or sticks of incense. We are too far uptown to feel the effects. We are too far away to see the people.

I call home. I have the irrational fear that someone from my family is down there, in all the smoke and fire. My little sister may have been on a field trip to the World Trade Center. My parents both work downtown. Were they scheduled to be there today? I cannot remember. I call again and again. Each time, the lines are busy.

It has been decided that we are to take one last surgical case for today before all elective cases are canceled. The hospital has been placed on crisis alert. Throughout the adult and children's hospitals, all but the sickest are being cleared from the ERs and ward beds. Beds are being shifted in the ICUs to make room for the wounded. We move through our last case in a daze, an orchiopexy on a five-year-old boy to bring down an undescended testicle into his scrotum. As his parents leave the OR after the induction of general anesthesia, it seems like they want to tell us something, but instead they just silently leave the room, one behind the other. I do not blame them for being concerned. Aside from the standard worries of any parent whose child is having surgery, who wants their child to be intubated on an OR table when, for all we know, the world is burning down around us?

The nurse bursts in one last time. "They collapsed. The Towers collapsed." And of course, I don't believe her.

Our final patient is wheeled to the Recovery Room, and we're back in the anesthesia conference room, watching footage of the Towers collapsing again and again and again, like images in a flip book. "People were jumping out of the windows," one of the anesthesiologists says, almost to herself. I walk by the Urology Department, see Dr. Harris sitting at the desk in his office alone. News updates are playing on the radio. He is sitting with his head in his hands.

Bob and I go back up to the tenth-floor skybridge. The smoke is still there, but the Towers are gone.

The hospital is on high alert. Overhead pages are

being issued with instructions of briefing meetings, and the halls are filled with people. Everyone, from attendings to residents to medical students, has been assigned a duty. We are scared, but reassured with a sense of purpose. *We can help! We can save! We can do something!* There is a sign-up desk in a room adjacent to the hospital cafeteria, where med students are to leave their names, pager numbers, and a list the first-aid techniques they are qualified to perform. Of course I lie a little, telling them that I can draw blood and start IVs, though as a fresh third-year med student, the only blood I've ever drawn has been off another med student's willingly pronated arm in a practice session, and the only IV I've ever placed has been in the sclerotic, multiply punctured vein of a disembodied, plastic mannequin hand. But I want so much to be able to help, so I tell them that I have the expertise. *This,* I feel, *is what I came to medical school to do.*

I call home, finally get through. My dad is fine, at home. My sisters are both at school, one on the Upper East Side, one at college in Massachusetts. My mom is at work, in Chinatown, near the epicenter of the chaos. I order her over the phone to stay at her office until things outside calm down, stay off the streets, deal with the problem of how to get home later. I pray that she listens to me, just for once. I am so thankful to hear their voices. I am so wildly thankful to *have* them, to know that they are well, and alive, on a day when so many are not, and all else seems uncertain. I make a mental note to, in the future, be more grateful for these small things, these assumed tautologies. *My family is alive. No one has hurt them.*

In the hospital everything is chaos. Local people from all over the neighborhood are pouring into the lobby, wanting to give blood, wanting to donate time, wanting to help, help, help. The only thing missing is patients. Due to our location at the far northern end of Manhattan island, we may be the New York hospital farthest away from the Financial District, and as we listen to the radio, hearing requests from Saint Vincent's, a small community hospital in Greenwich Village—*could any doctors with experience in trauma or plastic surgery please come down to our ER, we need extra hands*—we groan. We have the resources—our hospital is huge—but there's just no way we can get down to where we are needed.

The city is on terror alert. All highways to and from the hospital are closed to civilian traffic. Some people jump on bikes, get rides with police, and go downtown anyway. I walk by the orthopedics conference room and see residents standing shoulder to beefy shoulder, each one in a line popping antibiotics one after the other. If bioterrorism is the next strike, they want to be ready.

I meet up with a few students in the lobby of the medical school and we walk outside together. The day is dazzlingly bright, and up in our neighborhood, everything is surprisingly normal. People are walking out on the street. Businesses are open as usual. Even the coffee carts, with their waxy rows of doughnuts and rolls, are still working the sidewalks. The only clue that things are any different is the police barricades on either side of the block outside the ER, keeping the roads to the ambulance bay open in case any casualties should be sent our way. We run over to the bagel shop to grab something to eat. We want to be ready when the patients start coming up.

Back inside, we walk up to the surgical floor, and Mayor Giuliani is speaking on television. He tells us that in the end, the losses from the tragedy will be "more than we can bear." He looks shaken. He looks like he's ready to cry. I am too.

I find Joe wandering through the halls of the hospital, looking as lost as I feel, and we walk down to the Emergency Room together. Down on the first floor, the ER is packed, but for once, not with patients. Attendings, residents, and interns from all fields fill every corner of the room and sit in watchful wait. Waiting for the injured. Waiting to help. We have been instructed to stay uptown, to stay at our own hospital where we can be of most use. *Downtown is chaos,* we hear. *We would only be aggravating the situation by trying to head downtown.* We're taking what we've been told is the most helpful and constructive course of action. So why do we all feel so impotent?

Over the phone, over the radio, we hear about the situation from other hospitals. Saint Vincent's and NYU are busy, but farther uptown, Roosevelt has yet to receive any patients, and St. Luke's hasn't heard from anyone either. A good fifty blocks north of St. Luke's, we continue to wait. A measured voice can be heard from across the ER through the hush, one of the internal medicine attendings who has been coordinating some of the organizational efforts: "We're not going to get anyone up here today. Anyone who survived all that is going to be too critical to tolerate a half-hour ambulance ride up here. We may get some transfers for surgery after they're stabilized. But not today."

And so we keep waiting.

And waiting.

It's 7:00 p.m. and still, no one has come up from the rubble that in days to come will be known as "Ground Zero." A resident comes over to our gaggle of huddled medical students and gently encourages us to go home, they'll page us if they need assistance later on. *We live just across the street,* we tell him, *so we can get here in just a few minutes, just page us, let us know if there's any way we can help. We really want to help.* The resident is silent and then looks around. Except for the staff, the ER looks like a ghost town. There are no miraculous pulls from the rubble for us to work on, no casualties for us to bandage and splint, so that in doing our work, we can quiet the aching sadness in our own heads that such a thing could happen, that any plot could be so diabolical; there is nothing for us to temper the magnitude of all that suffering, and we were not able to be there for those who needed us. There are simply too few survivors to save. What good are doctors without patients to take care of?

We walk home slowly together, silently, and the sun is setting. The ambulance bay is empty and waiting, as it will continue to be all night.

Jeanne

In some ways being a medical student is one of the most difficult roles in the hospital. You are negotiating within an elaborate maze in which all the walls are invisible. *What should I be doing? Where should I stand? Is this the time to ask questions? If I step up now, will it be construed as inappropriate or overly aggressive? If I don't step up now, will I come off as passive and uninterested? What are my responsibilities and where are the boundaries? What should I be doing* right now?

I am halfway through my third year of medical school, deep in those dark months of the winter when you arrive at the hospital before sunrise and leave well after sunset, the days so dark and so cold that you feel as though daylight is maybe just a fanciful invention by Madison Avenue executives, concocted to sell sunglasses.

I am on my Neurology rotation at a cash-poor city hospital, which gives me new appreciation for the luxuries we unwittingly enjoy at Columbia-Presbyterian uptown. It is the first time this year that we as third-year medical students are being called on to act as junior residents—not necessarily because of our knowledge and experience but simply because the hospital needs the manpower. And it isn't just staff or medical equipment that is lacking—one day I spend twenty minutes wandering the wards just looking for a blank sheet of paper. "Is there any copier paper I could use?" I finally ask the ward clerk, whom I fortuitously catch three minutes after her coffee break and seven minutes before her next coffee break.

"No paper, we're out. We've been using this." And she leads me to a box of old expired nursing triplicate forms. "We don't use these anymore, so you can make copies on here." She flips over the forms and helpfully points out, "They're blank on the back." Not wanting to argue, I feed the triplicates into the paper rack and push the green button, but the paper jams in the ancient copier and now that's broken too. Just like half of the computers on the floor and the nursing intercom system and the lightbox down the hall, which forces us to hold up all our X-rays and CT scan printouts to the buzzing fluorescent lighting overhead, squinting to see the details.

This particular evening, I admit Jeanne, a thirty-six-year-old woman from the neighborhood who apparently had a massive stroke, to the inpatient Neurology service. She was making dinner at home when she suddenly collapsed. Her twelve-year-old daughter called the ambulance.

The most frustrating thing about Neurology is the fact that our understanding of the underpinnings of neurological disease so far vastly outstrips our ability to actually treat our patients. For so many of the stroke patients we admitted that month, we would spend hours talking about the patients' presenting symptoms, their residual neurological deficits, going over our neuroanatomy and pinpointing exactly what vessels, which areas, which nerve tracts had been knocked out. We would look at the CT scans. We would whip out our little reflex hammers, the Neurology residents would bring out all their little toys (they had the *best* toys)—ask patients to name objects, remember words, draw patterns, identify the smell of coffee grounds or peppermint from little jars they carried around with them. And then...aspirin. We would put these patients on aspirin, tell them that sometimes with time these deficits could improve (probably a small consolation to a seventy-eight-year-old man), and send them home after a few days. *Aspirin?* I think to myself. *Why even come into the hospital? I have aspirin at home.*

There are two differences with Jeanne. One is that at thirty-six, she is young compared to most stroke patients. Secondly, she arrived at the hospital within an hour of her stroke. For a variety of reasons, many stroke patients linger at home for hours, sometimes even days, before getting to a hospital. But for patients with the good fortune to present to us early, there are actual interventions that we may be able to perform that can sometimes reverse the damage of the stroke before the affected regions of the brain choke off and die.

Ischemic strokes are caused by decreased blood flow—and therefore decreased oxygen delivery—to discrete areas of the brain, usually caused by blood clots in the brain's circulation. The brain, an exquisitely sensitive organ, can tolerate only a few minutes without oxygen, after which time, brain tissue will start to die, leading to the impairments that we associate with strokes—numbness, weakness, inability to talk, confusion. Within a certain window of time, however, the clots causing these ischemic strokes can actually be dissolved by a delicate procedure using an agent known as tissue plasminogen activator (tPA); a small catheter is threaded through an artery in the patient's groin up into the blocked brain vessel. The goal is to restore blood flow to the ischemic brain regions before the damage becomes permanent. However, as with all things, there are certain criteria for the administration of tPA. Patients have to have a CT scan of the head to rule out a hemorrhagic stroke —bleeding into the brain tissue—as the administration of tPA in this situation could clearly make the bleed worse. By the same token, patients cannot have any other conditions that may predispose them to bleeding—recent surgery, low platelets, or the like. Finally, and perhaps most crucially, patients receiving tPA thrombolysis for ischemic stroke must receive treatment within three hours of the onset of symptoms. Which is why my resident and I are in the ER tonight, agitating for Jeanne's CT scan to be done, so we will have enough time to read it, rule out a bleed, and emergently transfer her uptown to Columbia so that the interventional neuroradiologist might actually be able to make her the one stroke patient this month whom we are able to save.

My resident, Dave, a small, compact man who looks like the personification of a Woody Allen movie, is not one to mince words. "Fucking *idiot*!" He is referring to the radiologist on call tonight, who refuses to clear space in the CT scanner for Jeanne. The radiologist's argument is that he is starting a scan on a patient in the ER to rule out appendicitis. It has now been two hours since Jeanne collapsed, and her time for intervention is running out. My resident argues, calls our attending, the chair of the department, anyone to step in, but the radiologist will not budge. *I'm taking care of an emergency too,* he argues. Time inexorably ticks by.

Four and a half hours after her daughter calls the ambulance, Jeanne finally gets her head CT. The stroke is not hemorrhagic, but the time window has closed. She does not get transferred to Columbia and she does not get tPA.

Up on the Neurology floor late that night, I am finishing my admission exam, getting Jeanne settled into her room (which, as the other bed is empty, is thankfully a single for now), tying up whatever loose ends I can manage before heading home for the night. Jeanne is sleepy, her voice slurred, the right side of her face sagging from the stroke. She asks me something indistinct, and, not understanding, I ask her to repeat the question.

"Am…I…going…to die?" she asks, looking straight at me. This is the first patient who has asked me this question. I have never had a patient die before, and the very concept is utterly alien to me. Why would she die? She is thirty-six years old. She is in the hospital now. We are taking care of her.

"No," I tell her firmly, not a strategy of bedside manner or just a reassuring answer before leaving for the night. I tell her she is not going to die because, with all the force of my youthful optimism and inexperience pressing down on me, I literally cannot conceive of the alternative.

* * *

Over the following week, I come to learn more about Jeanne, in that detached way that clinicians become acquainted with their patients without actually having ever known them outside of their illness. I meet her fiancé, Donnell, who keeps calling me "Doctor" despite my repeated corrections. As the medical student on the team, I am really more of a conduit for the flow of information than anything else, reporting on Jeanne's physical exam, lab results, medication list to the team on rounds, then parroting back the team's assessment and plan to Jeanne and Donnell, who hang on to every word. Our current hypothesis is that Jeanne may have some sort of rheumatologic disorder thus far undiagnosed, an autoimmune syndrome like lupus that may have predisposed her to forming blood clots, which led her to have a stroke at such a young age. Of course the blood work that would confirm such a diagnosis—more sophisticated tests that need to be sent off to an outside lab—is still pending, so there is little to tell Donnell when he comes by each day, hungry for news. So I just repeat the same things over and over again, feeling impotent. Donnell, a sad but pleasant bear of a man, is unflaggingly grateful for any news.

I learn some things about Jeanne and Donnell in this brief time. I learn that they have been together for five years. That they love basketball. They like to go to Madison Square Garden to watch the Knicks play when they get the chance. Sometimes they share a tub of popcorn. Donnell talks occasionally about Jeanne's daughter, the one who was with her when she had her stroke, and how she is holding up with her mother in the hospital. I never learn the daughter's name. I never ask.

Donnell comes by every evening after work. He helps Jeanne brush her teeth, wipes the saliva and toothpaste that leaks from the flaccid right side of her mouth. He helps Jeanne comb her hair. He holds her hand and tells her that things are going to be all right, even though it isn't clear that they will be. One morning, when I come in on rounds, there is a little note sitting on her meal tray to the left of her bed. It is signed, *"All my love, Donnell."* Quietly, without waking her, I move the note over to the right side of her bed—because of the stroke, she can no longer see anything on her left side.

But Jeanne is only one patient of several I am following that month, and as much as I would like to spend more time with her, I have other responsibilities, other people who I am helping to take care of as well. I am in one such other's room now, a twenty-four-year-old man with probable viral meningitis, when a nurse comes to find me. "She's complaining that her chest hurts," she tells me.

"Who's 'she'?" I ask, shining a light into the eye of my other patient. He winces and pushes my hand away, hissing *damn* under his breath.

"Room Eight," she replies, and she has my attention now. Jeanne's room. "They're in a meeting," she answers my next question before I ask—my resident is upstairs, in his weekly conference with the department chair. Hastily excusing myself, I rush down the hall to Jeanne's room.

It does not take three years of medical school

to determine that something is clearly wrong, very very wrong. Jeanne is breathing fast—panting would be a more accurate description—and, seeing me, lifts her good hand up to her sternum. "Hurts," she slurs. *Oh shit.*

Some of the other medical students are in the room now, having seen me rush down the hall. "Page Dave," I tell one of them, meaning our senior resident. "Tell him we need him in here now. And..." My mind is racing. What else should we do? Chest pain? Was she having a heart attack? *Heart attack.* "We probably should get the EKG machine in here."

Dave rushes in just as we are putting on the last of the EKG leads on and trying to get a clean strip. Like the rest of the equipment in this hospital, the EKG machine is old, really ancient, the kind where the leads attach to the patient's chest with conductive jelly and suction cups instead of stickers, and it is taking three medical students just to figure out how to turn the damn thing on. Jeanne heaves and repeats through her oxygen mask that *it hurts, chest hurts.*

We catch Dave up on the story and watch as his face darkens. One of my classmates tears off the EKG printout and whips out his calipers, a compasslike tool used to measure intervals on electrocardiograms, found solely in the pockets of cardiologists and overly earnest medical students. However, not having any really good sense of what to do with the results in this, an actual emergency, he thrusts the printout toward Dave, and we all pore over it.

I have not yet become proficient in interpreting the many jagged lines of the standard twelve-lead

EKG and am still laboriously trying to calculate Jeanne's heart rate and rhythm when Dave highlights the crucial points. "Here," he indicates, "and here," pointing to some abnormal patterns in the right-sided leads. "Tachy. Right heart strain."

"Does it look like she's having an MI?" I ask, meaning a myocardial infarction, the medical term for a heart attack.

"It's possible, but it looks more likely that she just had a massive PE." A pulmonary embolus, or a blockage of an artery in the lung, can often be caused by blood clots, usually originating from veins in the lower extremities. Like a stroke in the lung, a big enough blood clot can cause bleeding, cardiovascular collapse, even sudden death. *Of course.* It all makes sense—a patient who we believed to be predisposed to forming blood clots, a patient who already had a stroke, and who had been lying basically immobilized in bed for the better part of a week was a prime candidate for a PE. She was already on blood thinners after the stroke, of course, but it appears now that our current measures may not have been aggressive enough.

Things are moving quickly. Jeanne is readied for transport and rushed down for another CT scan, this time of her lung, to diagnose pulmonary embolism. She then goes straight from the CT scanner to the Intensive Care Unit, where she is started on an anticoagulant drip, where more lines and monitors are attached, and where every blip of her heart, or variation of her blood pressure, is broadcast on monitors out in the main nursing station. After she is up in the ICU, where the team falls upon her like mechanics at a pit stop in the Indy 500, Dave turns to all of us and pats me on the shoulder. "Nice job, guys. Good pickup." I want to protest that all we really did was come to the basically mindless realization that there was something wrong and wheel in the EKG machine—but decide to stay silent, because Dave is just being a nice guy, who realizes that words of affirmation for third-year med students are few and far between.

A few hours later, after things have settled down a little, I go visit Jeanne in the ICU. Donnell is there, of course, holding her hair, which seems a little strange until I realize that this is the only part of her body not tied down to some manner of monitoring or access line. The sharp, violent smell of urine hits me, and I realize that in all the time since the stroke, Jeanne has never been incontinent until today. Donnell looks at me, unsmiling and haggard, and in that moment I can see that the small, hopeful light in his eyes has dimmed.

This is the ICU, no longer the neurology ward, so I am tentative, my role here unclear. But I tell Donnell and Jeanne what happened, what we did, and what the different colored lines on the monitor are measuring. "She may stay here for a little while, getting stabilized, and then later, maybe she'll come back down to the neurology floor." Donnell nods slowly and says, "Thanks again for everything you've done, Dr. Michelle." Jeanne herself has not acknowledged that I am even in the room, and she stares off at a point on the wall somewhere behind my head. But as I watch, a tear leaks out the side of one eye and tracks down to her pillow.

I do not see Jeanne again. The life of a third-year medical student is nomadic by nature, and a few days after her transfer to the ICU, my five-week Neurology rotation is over and it is time for me to move on. I am sent off to Connecticut for five weeks to rotate through an affiliate hospital on Family Medicine, seeing toddlers with croup and middle-aged construction workers for Workman's Comp physicals. But at a medical school party about a month afterward, I bump into my classmate Amresh, who I know started his Neurology rotation through the same city hospital immediately after we left. "Hey, do you know whatever happened with that patient? Jeanne Thompson? Thirty-six-year-old lady? Had a stroke, then a PE?"

He frowns, scouring his memory. "Oh *right*. I remember her. She died a while ago, just a couple days after we came on service."

"She *died*?" I can't believe what I was hearing. "How could she die?" I mean to say how *did* she die, but somehow I guess it comes out wrong.

"Had another big PE." He pauses to take a drink from his cup. "Strange thing is that the lab stuff finally came back," referring to the original labs we had sent to look for any coagulation abnormalities, "and everything was normal. So we're not really sure why it all happened. Weird, huh?"

"Yeah," I answer, my mind reeling. "Weird." I think back to that first night that I admitted her, the time window for tPA that we missed. Would she have had a PE if she hadn't been paralyzed from her stroke? Would she have had a PE anyway? I think about what she had asked me that first night, and how I had completely brushed aside the question. *Pffft, you're not going to die. No one's going to* die *around here.* What was worse, the fact that I told her the lie, or the fact that I hadn't known any better than to believe it?

"You didn't *lie* to her," Joe points out to me later, as I rehash the story again and again. "You told her what you thought was true. Anyway, what were you *supposed* to say? 'Yes, you're going to die of a massive PE'? You said what you had to say, you said what you thought was the truth. You couldn't *know*."

I'm not really sure what the right answer to this question is, or if there *is* a right answer, but I know that I feel guilty somehow, and responsible. Maybe because she was young. Maybe because she had a daughter. Maybe because her fiancé was always so nice to her, and to me. Maybe because I had called her home once during her hospitalization, trying to reach Donnell for the answer to some question or other, but instead got her answering machine message. *"Hi, this is Jeanne,"* and you could hear the smile and energy in that voice, the contrast between that Jeanne and the Jeanne that lay in the bed in Room 8 so sharp that I winced. *"I can't answer your call right now, but leave a message, and I'll promise to call you back. God bless you, and have a great day."*

Decisions

It is March of my third year of medical school, and I have just started my Family Medicine rotation. The month-long rotation takes place at a community hospital in Connecticut, far enough away from Columbia that housing for students is provided adjacent to the hospital, in a strip of tenement housing made up of one-bedroom apartments, each equipped with a small kitchenette, TV, bed, bath, and whatever miscellaneous detritus the last student left behind. The first day of my rotation, I walk into the living room of my assigned apartment to see a sagging recliner pulled up within two feet of the TV, both sitting dead center in the otherwise bare room, the imprint of the other student's body still visible on the tacky upholstery. Spilled on a milk crate next to the recliner are a handful of change, a few packages of Saltines (no doubt purloined from the hospital), and a phone number for the car service company commissioned to shuttle med students to and from different hospital sites. It all looks deeply depressing.

Luckily, Joe and I have worked it out so that we are completing our Family Medicine rotation together, and we decamp into one single apartment, making it as livable as we can for our month in exile. The apartment has temperamental plumbing, few basic supplies, and no heat, so we improvise where we can, scurrying back and forth across the street to the hospital for what we need. We borrow blankets from the supply room in the ER to survive the frost, steal napkins from the hospital cafeteria when the toilet paper runs out, and, using a combination of student meal tickets and free food provided by pharmaceutical reps hawking one product or another, we are able to cobble together three meals a day. It is one of those experiences that, in retrospect, may eventually be considered charming and romantic—though during those freezing flophouse nights, huddled together under the crushing weight of ten scratchy hospital blankets and contemplating whether it would be worth it to keep the oven on overnight just for the heat it would provide, romance is the furthest thing from our minds.

Besides, we have bigger things to think about. Within the next few weeks, the third-year class is to submit rotation request forms for our fourth and final year of medical school, requests which, in theory, should be directed by the field of medicine we have decided to pursue. A student interested in pursuing a General Surgery residency, for example, would register to do several intensive surgical rotations early on in the summer and fall, perhaps also squeezing in rotations in the Intensive Care Unit and Emergency Room for good measure. Though no one pays much attention to rotations in the latter part of the year (there is a "senior spring" phenomenon in medical school too, where fourth-year students basically blow off the last few months of training, padding their schedules with cushy rotations in Dermatology or Radiology, sometimes doing rotations in exotic locations abroad, using the coursework as an excuse for travel), the construct of the first few months of fourth year is vitally important. We have to decide which rotations we need to do, but before we do that, we have to decide what kind of doctors we want to be. I am still stuck on the latter.

"How are we supposed to *know* already?" I

protest. "We haven't even finished third year yet, and already we have to commit to one thing? We still have a ton of rotations to go! We haven't even rotated through General Surgery yet! How am I supposed to know whether or not I want to do one of those things when I haven't even tried them?"

"I don't know," Joe answers. "What should *I* do? What do you think? Emergency Medicine?" His sister is an ER nurse in inner-city Baltimore and seems to enjoy her work, or at the very least enjoys the effect of relaying her more shocking or grotesque war stories whenever she gets a chance.

"I have no idea. I haven't done an ER rotation yet either. Seems a little chaotic for me, though."

"Well," continues Joe, "what about Pediatrics? Weren't you all lathered up about that after your Peds rotation this fall?"

"Well, yeah, but now I'm getting cold feet. I mean, yes, *literally* my feet are cold." I gesture to our sad hospital housing, where outside frost is caked on the windows, and inside we can see our own breath. "But I mean—what if I don't want to be treating snotty noses and writing prescriptions for amoxicillin my whole life? What if I want to do something less office-based, more procedure-based? What if I even want to do something surgical?"

"Then do that."

"Or what about something like Ob-Gyn? That has clinical medicine *and* surgery. That could be interesting. Except—oh my god, what am I saying? Did I just say that I might want to go into *Ob-Gyn*? All those screaming ladies and yeast infections and nights on call in Labor and Delivery for the rest of my life? After I had that one Ob-Gyn attending tell me point blank that I should never, ever, *ever* go into Ob-Gyn because that's what he did and he was miserable? Help me. I don't know what I want to do."

"Look," Joe says logically. "Let's make a list. Write down generally what it is that you want to do with your life and with your career before you get too specific. Then you can narrow it down at least."

"OK." I consider the basics. "I want to be a doctor who works directly with patients every day, so not Pathology or anything like that. I would like to do *some* procedures, though I don't need to be doing procedures all day every day or anything." I thought some more. "I want...I want to have a *life.* I don't want to live like a med student forever. I want to have a family, and I want to have time to spend with them. I want to *enjoy* my work but I want to be *able* to enjoy it because I have the ability to leave the hospital sometimes. I don't need to make a whole lot of money, but I want to be able to, you know, send my kids to school and, you know, live comfortably." I pause. "Oh, and I don't want to go into any field where the other doctors are assholes. I want to work with people who are nice." I look hopefully at Joe. "So, what do we have?"

"Well, so far you just ruled out Pathology and Cardiothoracic Surgery. I think everything else is still on the table."

"Shit." I flip through the course catalog, look over the rotation offerings in Pediatric Otolaryngology, Geriatric Medicine, Neuroradiology. So many choices, so many directions to go. Can it be possible that any-one in our class *really* knows what kind of doctor they want to be already? How are we equipped to make this decision at this point? What do we really know about medicine, or even about what we want?

"What about you?" I ask Joe. "What about *your* wish list?"

"About the same as yours," he answers. "Don't worry, we don't have to decide right now."

"No, not right now. Just three weeks from now. That's plenty of time to figure out our whole lives, right?"

"Sure. Plenty of time."

Turns out a big piece of the puzzle falls into place sooner than that. A few days later, during a weekend visit back to New York, Joe and I are having dinner together when, with no prelude, he reaches into his jacket pocket and pulls out a small, black velvet box.

"So look, I was wondering," he says, almost busi-nesslike, as if he were on the wards presenting a potential treatment plan that he wants me to eval-uate, "if you wouldn't mind, you know, being my wife."

I smile. "No, I guess I wouldn't mind that too much." Some decisions are easier than others.

Sink or Swim

It is July again, and I am now a fourth-year medical student on my subinternship in Pediatrics. After tor-turing myself with weeks more of indecision the pre-vious spring, I finally decided to apply for a residency in Pediatrics, mostly because I honestly enjoy Pediatric medicine, but also just to commit to *something* so that I can move on with my life. Joe meanwhile decided at the last possible moment to apply for a residency in Ophthalmology, a choice that seemed to come out of nowhere, though the more I learn about the field, the more I think it seems uniquely suited to his temperament. As it turns out, Joe is a perfect fit for this surgical subspecialty valuing academia, precision, and a meticulous attention to detail, and is himself starting a subinternship at the Harkeness Eye Institute.

A subinternship, or "sub-I" (as it is known to those of us who cannot get through a sentence without an acronym or abbreviation) is basically the training bra of residency. It is a prerequisite for graduation from medical school, consisting of a month where we assume the patient load and care responsibilities of a first-year resident (or "intern"), albeit with the increased supervision and support required by logic and law. It is a dress rehearsal for the real thing.

In one sense, being a sub-I is the logical progression from being a third-year medical student. *See one, do one, teach one* is one oft-repeated credo of academic medicine, and after a year of watching residents in action, it seems due time for us to start "doing" on our own. Sounds reasonable enough. However, the reality of the transition from third-year med student to sub-intern is more like being lifted dripping from a knee-deep wading pool in which beach balls and foam noodles lazily float, and thrown headfirst into the churning ocean, with only these instructions to guide you: *keep your head above water and try not to die.*

"How do you *do* it?" I asked my intern once when I was a third-year medical student. I was watching her juggle twenty-five patients, a ceaseless stream of urgent pages, three simultaneous emergencies, all while drinking a full cup of coffee without spilling a drop. She had at this point been awake for the past twenty-seven hours.

"You just *do it*," she answered cryptically, one-handedly typing a note into the computer while picking up the phone to answer her latest page. At the time, I didn't really understand this philosophy, which I had heard from several other residents before—chalked it up as one of those nonsensical sayings like, "It is what it is," stemming from a culturally saturating Nike ad campaign. But when I started my sub-I—started being on the receiving end of those endless pages, the first person called in an emergency, realizing that for the first time, I was not simply a passive observer or an extra set of hands but actually *responsible* for these patients under my care—I got it. *You just do it.* You can't think about how much there is to do, or how much is going on, or how tired you are. There's no time for that. So you just *do it.* You put your head down and get to work, and at the end of the night you look up and realize that you got through it all. And then you go home and come back the next morning and do it again. This is what I am learning from my sub-I. I am learning that I can do this.

Most of the time.

Right now, I am trying to draw blood from one of my patients, Jacob, a seven-year-old boy with a mysterious case of hepatitis. So far, preliminary tests have for the most part ruled out infection or a drug-mediated cause of his liver inflammation, but we still cannot explain his skyrocketing liver function tests or the fact that he is so jaundiced that he has actually crossed the threshold from yellow to faintly glowing neon green. He lies there in bed, looking like a tennis ball, while I wipe down the inside of his elbow, looking for veins.

My first successful blood draw on a patient was during my Internal Medicine rotation in third year. My resident, appalled that I had never been given the chance, took me into the room of one of his patients, a comatose eighty-two-year-old woman who'd been sent in from a nursing home with a fever. "Here's a good one for you to try!" he said cheerfully, producing all of the necessary equipment and bottles from the pocket of his lab coat like a magician. And while I felt a little ghoulish, taking advantage of an unfortunate situation, she *was* a good patient to try on. The patient required blood cultures, entailing not one but *two* blood draws, each from a separate site. (I ended up getting the second sample from the top of her foot.) She didn't care that I was a medical student, never uttered a word of protest, and most importantly, didn't move a muscle.

Subsequent to that, I have drawn blood a number of times on patients, some considerably more alert, but never on a child. Most of my phlebotomy has been confined to adults, who have the two important qualities of being larger (with, crucially, larger veins to hit) and more obedient. You take out a needle in front of an adult and ask them not to move, and for the most part, the adults will not move. Take out a needle in front of a child, especially a seven-year-old child, and chances are that you will need two or three people to hold him down. I have already enlisted the boy's mother and nurse for this task. My senior resident stands back by the door, unobtrusively supervising me and perhaps positioning herself to catch Jacob in the event that he bolts.

The most difficult part for a novice drawing blood is the actual point at which the needle breaks the skin. There is that ingrained taboo one has to overcome about jamming sharp objects through other people's flesh, and during my early attempts at drawing blood last year, my initial approaches with the needle merely dented the skin without actually pushing through it. "What the hell are you doing?" the intern supervising me for the procedure hissed. "I don't want to hurt him," I whispered back, at which time the intern pointed out that it was probably more painful for our patient to be gently prodded repeatedly by a 23-gauge needle rather than being swiftly pierced once and getting the damn thing over with. I try to keep these things in mind as I swipe Jacob's arm with an alcohol swab, hiding the butterfly needle behind my back, out of view.

Of course he is screaming already. Hiding the needle until the last second isn't fooling anyone: he knows the cues—tourniquet, the astringent smell of alcohol, his mother squashing down on his body like a sandbag. I figure that the emotional damage won't be minimized by any further glad-handing and, with a cheery voice, tell Jacob that he's going to feel a little bee sting. Do New York kids even *know* what a bee sting feels like? *I* certainly have never been stung by a bee. Why do I even say this?

I have envisioned a prolonged slog, fishing for invisible vessels through layers of fat, sawing back and forth through tissue planes as Jacob lies shrieking and flailing beneath me. But to my surprise, I hit the vein almost immediately. Is there anything more gratifying than seeing that thick maroon column rising up through the hub of the needle and the tubing? Is there any greater high for a medical student than to actually do a procedure cleanly and correctly? I am giddy with the thrill of achievement. After drawing off a syringe full of blood, I withdraw the needle and apply pressure to the venipuncture site with a square of clean gauze. "You were so brave," I tell Jacob, who has stopped screaming but stares at me with big watery eyes full of recrimination. Feeling that some elaboration is called for, I add, "As brave as He-Man."

He stares blankly at me. Realizing I am dating myself with pop-culture references to my own mid-1980s childhood, I scour my brain for a more timely children's cartoon character. *Brave as She-Ra? Brave as Lion-O from the Thundercats? Brave as Hefty Smurf?* Crap. What the hell do kids watch these days?

"Very brave," I repeat lamely. I lift up the gauze. The bleeding has stopped. I place a small round

Band-Aid over the site, and Jacob's mother, who is probably only in her late twenties though she looks much older from weeks of worry and fatigue, smiles and thanks me.

Exiting the room, my senior resident claps me on the shoulder. "Nice job with that blood draw. Now let's get it off to the lab before it clots."

"Right," I tell her, still practically levitating with a sense of accomplishment. I uncap the top of the test tube as I have seen other residents do, to avoid the risk of accidentally sticking myself with the needle during the transfer of blood from syringe to lab tubing. Squirting the blood into the glass vial, I tell her, "I'll have transport pick it up right now." But as I attempt to press the lid back on the test tube, something happens, some slippage or fumble, and somehow, I'm not quite sure how, I end up absolutely covered with Jacob's blood. I look like Carrie at the prom, minus the telekinesis and murderous rage.

My senior steps in, grabs what's left of the test tube before I manage to spill it, and peers inside. "There's still enough in here for them to run the sample. Why don't I take care of this? You"—she looks at me, a performance art version of Jackson Pollock, still speechless with disbelief—"should probably clean up a little."

One of my classmates, also on her Pediatrics sub-I, approaches me with a handful of individually wrapped alcohol swabs. "You should probably wash with soap after this," she says, ripping open one and dabbing at my chest, "but we can get off most of it with the wipes." A few third-year medical students come over and get in on the act, blotting at my arms, my hands, my back. How the hell did blood get on my *back*? Did I actually just take the tube of blood and *pour* it over my head? I feel ridiculous, but still, it must be noted, my overwhelming mood is still pride for having drawn the blood at all. As my classmates tend to me, I think to myself that we must look, from a distance, like a family of chimps, grooming one wayward member of the clan who doesn't have enough sense to keep herself clean and out of trouble.

* * *

It is two thirty in the morning, and I am watching a baby suffocate.

Taisha is a three-month-old girl who was admitted earlier today with bronchiolitis, a viral infection that can cause inflammation, increased mucous secretion, and plugging of the small airways delivering oxygen to the lungs. Affected patients can present with wheezing, increased work of breathing, and decreased oxygen in the blood, occasionally requiring supplemental oxygen or even mechanical ventilation of the lungs. And indeed, this is exactly how Taisha came to us. She was admitted from the Emergency Room wheezing, breathing fast, with an oxygen saturation of 93 percent (healthy patients usually measure 97 to 100 percent). We started her on supplemental oxygen via nasal cannula, short plastic tubing that fed into her nose, placed on a continuous pulse oximeter to measure her oxygen saturation, and ordered for close respiratory checks throughout the night. I have been coming by her room every hour or two to check her respiratory effort, her oxygen saturation, the rate of breathing, and to listen to the movement of air in her tiny chest.

Or, in this case, the lack thereof. Taisha is breathing quickly, grunting, her ribs and clavicles clearly visible as her tiny muscles pull and fight for each hard-won breath. Through my stethoscope, her lungs sound closed off, crackly. Her oxygen saturation is down to 88 percent. Whatever we are doing is not working.

The problem with bronchiolitis is that secretions and inflamed tissue plug the small airways. The more airways that are plugged, the less of the lung is available for oxygen exchange, and unless some measure is taken to stent open these airways, the patient breathes harder and harder to compensate, eventually tiring out and going into respiratory failure. This is what we are seeing with Taisha. She is breathing at an astronomical rate, almost eighty breaths per minute. She is not going to be able to sustain this all night—at some point, we are going to have to help her breathe.

We try the easy things first: humidified breathing treatments, thinning and suctioning out her secretions, patting her chest in an attempt to open up the closed airways. This helps a little bit, and her oxygen saturation goes up to 90 percent, but still, we need to do more.

My senior resident, I know, is attending to another emergency two floors down. I don't know what he is doing or how long he is going to be, and I also know that we don't have that much time to wait. So I make a decision. I decide that we need to start Taisha on CPAP.

CPAP, which stands for continuous positive airway pressure, is a way to help stent open airways that would otherwise be collapsed. In children, it is applied much like a nasal cannula, with tubing through the nose, only instead of just providing extra oxygen, a continuous level of pressure is applied into the airways. Think of sticking your head out of a car while driving down the highway. CPAP helps patients breathe, but crucially, it does not take over the work of breathing for them as a ventilator would—the goal is to buy the patient some time and avoid intubation and mechanical ventilation, with its attendant airway trauma and complications, if at all possible. And CPAP can often—with this extra bit of pressure being enough to help open up the collapsed airways in infants with bronchiolitis—give the patient a little help to decrease the work of breathing against an uncooperative set of lungs.

I look around. This seems like one of those decisions that I would run by my resident—"Say, should we maybe think about starting CPAP on this patient?"—and that he would approve, thus confirming my instincts are correct. But there is no one for me to ask at this moment. Aside from the nurses, who cannot write orders on patients, I am the only medical professional on the floor, and I am acutely aware that I don't even have an MD to my name yet. What should I do? Should I keep calling my resident? I paged him once more a few minutes ago, but, caught up in some crisis, he hasn't been able to call me back yet. I peek in on Taisha one more time. She is struggling. Her oxygen saturation is down to 89 percent again. So I pick up the phone and page the respiratory therapists to set up the CPAP apparatus, with the option to escalate to BiPAP, or bi-level positive airway pressure, which instead of a continuous level of pressure provides two different levels of pressure for inhalation and exhalation. In a dire emergency, BiPAP can help, but if a patient is in true respiratory failure, it will only temporize the situation until we will ultimately need to intubate the patient, risking lung damage and infection.

It takes a little time for the respiratory therapists to answer, and when they finally call back, they put up a fight. "We're pretty swamped right now," one of them tells me, "one of our therapists called in sick tonight, and we just set up a ventilator in the ICU. Most of the BiPAP units are being used, we only have one left, do you really need it? Can you call back in twenty minutes?"

"No," I cut him off, and I am a little surprised at the tone of my voice, as I usually tend toward meek and deferential. "I need this CPAP set up, and I really need it now. We have a three-month-old with bronchiolitis satting eighty-nine percent on nasal cannula, breathing at eighty-five, retracting into her back. I need the CPAP up here in five minutes. Is there a supervisor or someone else I need to call to make this happen?"

Christ, I think to myself, *this had better be the*

right decision. I'm using up the last BiPAP setup, the
respiratory therapist is going to murder me for get-
ting uppity, and I'm starting noninvasive ventilator
support on this kid when I'm technically not even al-
lowed to write orders on my own yet. If I am making
the wrong decision right now, I'm definitely going
down with all guns blazing.

Seven minutes later, the respiratory therapist arrives. Once he gets to the floor, I fall over myself with
sweet talk, thanking him for his expediency, apologizing for my tone on the phone, and finally showing
him into Taisha's room, where her nurse is suctioning her out again, patting on her little heaving chest.
Once he sees the baby, the respiratory therapist starts
to move a little faster. "There's a kid who needs to be
on CPAP," he agrees, unwrapping the tubing and af-
fixing it to our oxygen supply.

We are getting settled when Chris, my senior resident, walks into the room. Having dealt with the
crisis downstairs, he is now returning all his missed
pages and checking in on all the juniors he is supervising for the night. I have no doubt that, being the
most junior of the juniors, I'm one of the first he's
coming to see.

He has already spoken to the nurse and is looking
slowly around the room, taking stock of the situation.
Is he angry that I didn't try harder to call him before
starting CPAP? Pissed because he doesn't agree with
my decision? Or am I so off the mark that this intervention is actually hurting Taisha more than it is
helping? "Well, I guess that settles it," he finally says.
"You're ready."

"Ready for what?" I am still a little distracted, listening to Taisha's chest, looking at her vitals on the monitor next to her bed. She is already doing better, her respiratory rate slowing down, her oxygen saturation improving.

"You're ready to be an intern."

The Match

Of all the years of medical school, fourth year seems to go by the quickest. There are the mandatory rotations, then the roster of electives, some intensive and others more akin to the film and sculpture classes you might have taken the spring semester of your senior year in college. But after three-and-a-half years of medical school, we all feel entitled to a little senior slump.

Other things are going on too. We are applying for residencies, taking our suits and heels out of mothballs, and hitting the road for another round of interviews. We visited many programs, considered many options. And finally, that March brings the day that will determine our futures, at least for the next few years—through the much-anticipated phenomenon known as The Match.

Applying for residencies in medicine is not like applying for a regular job, or even like applying for medical school. Rather, you as the applicant interview at X number of residency programs (which can vary anywhere from three to several dozen) and rank these programs in order of preference. Simultaneously, the various residency programs interview Y number of students and construct a list themselves, ranking these applicants in order of desirability. On a specific day, both the students and the programs submit their lists, some magical computer compares the two, crunches some numbers, divides by the square root of negative one, and attempts to place every student into the highest-ranked program that ranked that student. Most applicants get placed, some applicants don't. Those who don't rank have the option to frantically find an open spot, any spot, at some program, or alternatively wait it out and try The Match again next year. And year after year, so it goes. I never said it wasn't confusing.

The very nature of the beast is that The Match truly does "match" you with one program and one program alone, which you can either accept or decline to attend. For the most part, there are no fallback plans, no second choices. What The Match gives you, you need to accept, or risk not having a residency spot anywhere at all.

The matter of The Match for couples is particularly fraught. When two medical students enter The Match together—a husband-and-wife pair, for example—they risk the possibility that one member of the couple may Match in New York while the other may Match in Fargo, North Dakota. Fortunately, many have the option to "Couples Match," a process in which the two residency applications of the couple are essentially bound together, so that they Match as a geographical unit, even if one partner is applying in Orthopedics and the other is applying in Psychiatry. What usually ends up happening in this situation is that both members of the couple get geographically matched to the highest ranked program of the partner in the more competitive (and therefore more difficult to place) specialty. Which can theoretically create resentment and stress, because, *Look, I could have Matched at this awesome program in New York on my own, but now because of you, here we are, moving to Fargo. Where are my snow boots?*

Regardless, Joe and I are unable to participate in the Couples Match, even though we would have chosen to, because ophthalmology as a field has its own separate Match system. Depending on where he applies, and where I apply, there is a very real possibility that we could be Matched in two separate cities. Two separate states. Hell, possibly even opposite sides of the country. Needless to say, this would be suboptimal.

In trying to figure out how best to approach The Match, I encounter a shocking number of people who, despite knowing that we will be married by the time our residencies start, casually ask, "So, do you guys actually want to live in the same place?" It is a surprising question, though I understand why people are asking. I have heard of a few couples—committed to each other, even married ones—who purposely did their residencies in different locations so they could each train at the best programs possible, even if it meant living apart. In fact, there is a surgery resident right now—married with two children, his wife not even in the medical profession—who lives and works at Columbia in New York City while his wife and children remain in Michigan. Between being on call and working nights and almost every weekend, this surgery resident has a total of maybe fifteen days per year that he does not have to be at the hospital. I presume he sees his family then.

Joe and I are not OK with this arrangement. The idea of getting married and then spending the next three or four years living in separate cities is not something we are willing to consider. Over the past four years, we have invariably prioritized medical training above our own needs, but on this matter we refuse to budge. So our solution, rather than risk Matching in different cities, is to only rank programs in a *single* city, that city being New York.

This gambit is vastly more risky for Joe than for me—Pediatrics is a relatively noncompetitive Match, but Ophthalmology is much more cutthroat, and applicants usually rank as many programs as possible. However, Joe is a strong candidate and willing to chance it. And so on Match Day, we find that we have both Matched at our first-choice programs, I in a three-year Pediatrics residency at the Children's Hospital of New York, and Joe in the three-year ophthalmology program at Columbia, where he will start after completing a preliminary year of general medicine at Mount Sinai Hospital on the Upper East Side of Manhattan.

In April, Joe and I get married in a small ceremony in New York City. We have the reception at South Street Seaport, near the Financial District, with a view of the Brooklyn Bridge and the negative space where the Twin Towers would have, *should* have been. During the reception, I see more than one person looking out the windows toward downtown, and I can tell what they are thinking, the view that they are searching for in their minds. Where the Towers once stood is now just clouds, sun, and open sky. The rest of the evening passes in the glow of memories and possibility, surrounded by family and friends, all framed by an encroaching dusk punctuated by twinkling lights of the city skyline.

Afterward, Joe and I take a sixteen-day honeymoon to southern Italy, which we enjoy not just for the scenery and amazing food but because we both know that this will be the longest vacation we will be able to take for at least the next ten or fifteen years. In some sense, it is a honeymoon not just of our marriage, but also of our medical careers. Afterward will come graduation, residency, and all the work and responsibility that somehow we signed up for, but for these two weeks we relish the opportunity to not think about medicine at all, instead soaking in the sweet Mediterranean sunshine and stuffing ourselves full of pasta and cannoli. We arrive back in New York early in May, tanned and refreshed, and a few weeks later receive our medical degrees.

In contrast to all the images I've cultivated of this particular moment of my life, graduation from medical school is a distinct letdown. After Match Day and the wedding, it almost seems like an afterthought, a technicality. It is raining steadily throughout the day, and as we file through the courtyard to the tent in the back garden of the hospital, we are dodging raindrops and the pointy ends of umbrellas wielded by the various onlookers. A recorded processional is playing, not

"Pomp and Circumstance" like I had imagined, but something else in that genre, heavy on the brass. The tent erected over the graduation proceedings is sagging with the weight of accumulated rainwater, which unfortunately pools directly over the podium where the invited speaker, former *New York Post* columnist Jimmy Breslin, is giving his charge to the graduates. I will remember almost nothing of what he is saying to us, and more recall holding my breath, looking at the roughly thirty or so gallons of water sagging in a tarp reservoir over his head, wondering how much longer the structure will hold.

Finally, obligatory rhetoric dispensed, they call us up to the podium one by one to receive our diplomas. "Michelle Au, MD," the dean of students intones, handing me in a plain manila envelope what is probably one of the most important documents of my life. And then she is on to the next name. I wander off the stage and, unclear of where I should go next or what I should do, snake my way back through the audience to my seat. I look at my diploma, and there it is, my name in raised gothic script. *That's it?* I look up, see my other classmates, wandering about looking dazed, unsure. *After four years, that's all there is?* I don't know what exactly I expected—some feeling of crossing over, a dawning sense of expertise and maturity maybe, or at least some whispered secret from the old guard to the new. *Listen, we never told you this, but the secret to being a good doctor is this...* But there is none of that. We were now just 150 of the greenest doctors in the country, standing outside wearing our nice shoes in the rain.

What I realize some years later is this: going to medical school is like a wedding. Lots of work to be sure, but at many points interspersed with pomp and speeches and ceremony, moments highlighted and emphasized to scream THIS IS IMPORTANT, ultimately capped off with a walk down the aisle and hors d'oeuvres. Medical school is like the wedding, but being a doctor is like actually being married. And that's where the real hard work starts.

4 . PEDIATRICS

July

THE NIGHT BEFORE MY FIRST DAY of Pediatrics residency, I prepare everything for the following morning as meticulously as only a former med student who once employed a four-color note-taking system can. I have my new white coat (thrilling for its knee-skimming length—only medical students wear the short hip-length white coats, and I'm not a med student anymore, am I?) on a hanger by the door of our bedroom. The pockets of the coat are stuffed with all the things I think I will need tomorrow: Two pens. An antimicrobial reference guide. A spiral-bound pocket guide, *Spanish for Pediatrics*. My stethoscope and newly issued hospital pager. A small stash of brightly colored stickers for the children I will inevitably be torturing with my well-intentioned ministrations.

I take probably ten minutes fastidiously pinning and unpinning my name tag over the left chest pocket, trying to get it lined up perfectly straight. DR. MICHELLE AU, it declares unambiguously, in stark blue print. See, I'm a *doctor* now; even my name tag says so. They wouldn't have issued me a name tag if they didn't believe that I was capable of stepping up to the job, would they? Tomorrow, I will walk into the hospital, start taking care of my patients, and just like that, it will begin. I have graduated from medical school. *I am a doctor now.*

Then again, there is the small fact that I am absolutely scared to death.

Due to a purposely front-loaded schedule my fourth year of medical school, it has been five months since I have done anything even vaguely clinical, and ten months since I last saw a pediatric patient. I have a sneaking and not totally unsubstantiated fear that I have forgotten everything I ever learned about medicine.

Not that there is anything to do about that now. I set my bedside alarm clock for 4:00 a.m. Then I walk over to Joe's side of the bed and set the second alarm clock for 4:03 a.m. Just in case. Despite the fact that I don't think I will be doing anything approximating sleep that night, let alone risk oversleeping, I believe in the Boy Scout motto, *Be prepared.*

After brushing my teeth and fussing with my name tag one more time (it occurs to me that a carpenter's level or protractor might be of use here), I turn out my light at 9:45 p.m. and crawl into bed to commence six hours and fifteen minutes of staring at the ceiling. Over by the closet, my white coat hangs, illuminated by the light of the city filtering through our windows. Suspended over my scuffed clogs lined up underneath, the image it creates is that of an invisible doctor, standing silently and watching me sternly as I lie there in bed, helpless to do anything but stare back.

* * *

My decision to go into pediatrics was not straight-forward, though initially it seemed like it should be. *Hey, I like kids, kids like me, why the hell not.* I guarantee you that across the country, hundreds of small, female medical students are professing their desire to go into pediatrics, if only for the reason that it's one of the few fields where the patients are cute, smaller than us, and thus easily overpowered. True, I liked the idea of continuity of care, watching children grow up, and often being the doctor for not just the child, but the entire family—but really, I liked that pediatricians on the whole seemed sweet and nice and never yelled at me, even in my stupidest medical student moments. I did have my flashes of indecision of course, but in the end settled on pediatrics because, frankly, it seemed natural enough, and I had to do *something*, didn't I? Why pediatrics? Why *not*?

So now I am a Pediatrics resident. I have all the accoutrements of the well-intentioned Pediatrics intern: distracting toys, brightly colored Band-Aids, the ability to easily recover from a crouched position, and a ballpark familiarity with Pokémon or Pogs or whatever the hell else it is that kids like to play with these days. I walk into the room of my patient, the first patient of my fledgling pediatric career.

The patient is twenty-seven years old.

Joshua Vargas was born with chronic granulomatous disease, a disorder of certain white blood cells that renders them unable to destroy bacteria. Because of this, patients with CGD suffer from recurrent infections due to the impaired ability of their immune systems to fight them off. Usually these patients are admitted to the hospital with pneumonia or abscesses, though other types of skin, bone, or blood infections are common as well. Due to the nature of his disease, Josh has been in and out of the hospital since he was born, frequently requiring prolonged courses of antibiotic treatment to fight off the microbial scourge that his body cannot. He knows everyone here. He has been under his pediatrician's care for most of his life. The children's hospital, for better or worse, is his second home. When Josh turned twenty-one, he asked (perhaps demanded would be a better word) that his care not be transferred to the Infectious Disease specialists over at the adult hospital, but continue with his Pediatrics team. And while the good nature of his pediatricians accounted in some part for the accommodation of his request, I'm also sure that the adult doctors hadn't been thrilled with the prospect of inheriting a chronically ill patient with a medical chart that could be measured not in pages, but in pounds.

So for one reason or another, the administrators at the children's hospital agreed to look the other way.

Josh could continue to be admitted and receive care at the children's hospital, followed by his primary pediatrician, at least until future provisions could be made for his transfer of care. The only stipulation they made was that when Josh is admitted to the hospital, he is always given a single room. Due to his immunocompromise and the infectious nature of his disease, he probably would have been given a single anyway, but it seemed everyone wanted to avoid the awkwardness of having to room a twenty-seven-year-old man with a ten-month-old baby.

So this is how it comes to be that I am three years younger than my first Pediatrics patient.

I have done my homework, brushed up on his chart and the disease process, so at least I have something to grab on to. After knocking on the door, I walk into Josh's room, where he is lying in bed, watching a show on the dilapidated Zenith TV that hangs from the ceiling. He is thin and probably stands no more than 5'4'' tall, but is unmistakably an adult. "Josh, how are you?" He smiles pleasantly, accustomed to this morning routine. "My name is Michelle Au, I'm one of the doctors taking care of you today." While on the subway that morning, I had rehearsed in my head how I should introduce myself. Do I introduce myself as "Michelle," to be egalitarian, in a sort of, *We're buddies, you can tell me anything* kind of way? As "Dr. Au," to be clear about my role and inspire trust? Or should I go with the wordy introduction that I heard one of the senior Peds residents give a family once, one that left things open: "Hello, I'm Dr. Schweitzer, my first name is Audra, I'll be helping to take care of you today." Finally, I decided to go with the lead-in that made me most comfortable. I don't feel quite right introducing myself as "Dr. Au," not just yet. Like my new white coat, the title still feels too big.

"Hi," Josh answers. He waits for me to go on.

What am I supposed to say now? Do I go over his history again? Sit down? Wait for him to talk? A thousand options flash through my head, and I flip through these like a deck of cards before settling on something easy, to buy me some time. "How are you feeling today?"

"Fine. I'm good." Josh was hospitalized last week for a recurrent bout of bacterial pneumonia, for which he is currently receiving treatment. "Earlier this weekend was kind of bad, but since then I've been able to come off the face mask to nasal cannula. Yesterday I only needed two liters, and that was mostly for overnight." He indicates the oxygen port sticking from the wall, around which, sure enough, a length of plastic tubing is coiled.

"Great, great! That's...great." I think of what to say next. "Still coughing?"

"Not as bad. ID still wants another sputum culture to send off"—*ID?* I think. *What ID? My ID? Oh, he means the Infectious Disease team*—"so I'm trying to cough up something to give them." He lifts a sterile specimen cup sitting on his bedside tray and waggles it at me, like a man at a bar requesting a refill. Which, bizarrely, he is old enough to be.

"Sounds good." I flounder for a moment, then remember something from his chart to thrust at him, like a peace offering. "I saw that we were switching around some of your antibiotics last week."

"Yeah, after some of the sensitivities came back, Dr. Prince made some changes." He must be talking about the antibiotic sensitivities of the microbes they cultured. "And we got a new PICC in on Thursday, so I'm ready once they decide that I can go home." A PICC line, I remember, is a central line that can be placed for patients who need prolonged courses of IV antibiotic treatment. Unlike IVs, which must be changed every few days and which infiltrate easily, PICC lines can be kept in for several weeks. *What does PICC stand for anyway? Percutaneous...something...something...catheter? Oh shut up, it's not like he's going to ask. Peripheral...intravenous... shit. Gotta look that up.*

"Mind if I take a listen?" The stethoscope is something solid to grab on to and gives me a doctor-y thing to do. Josh, ever the obliging patient, sits up more and pulls up the back of his shirt. "Take some deep breaths," I tell him, but of course he doesn't need my prompting. He is a pro. His lungs sound coarse, crackly, and all this deep breathing on Josh's part triggers a chain of coughs. I briefly listen to his heart before pulling back down his shirt and patting him on the shoulder.

"I'll be back with the rest of the team later on," I tell him as he settles onto his pillow and turns his head back to the television. "Is there anything that I can get you for now? Some water?"

"No, I'm good. Thanks. My nurse is going to be in here soon anyway, I think it's time for my vanc."

Vanc? I think. *Oh, vancomycin. Antibiotic. Through his PICC line.* I am catching up. Josh smiles again. Really, he's a very nice boy. Or nice man, whatever.

"OK, I'll see you again in about two hours. Get some rest, and enjoy"—my eyes flick to the TV, where a screaming match is breaking out, and press-on nails are being ripped off in preparation for the oncoming melée—"the rest of *Jerry Springer.*" I wash my hands carefully at the sink and excuse myself.

Walking back down the hall to the nursing station, wiping down the bell of my stethoscope with an alcohol pad, I look shamefacedly down at my hands. *My first patient knows more about medicine than I do.*

* * *

It is Wednesday, two days into my internship, and another nurse is yelling at me.

I think there are several ways that nurses tend to deal with inexperienced young doctors. The first, and I think the nicest way, is to try to tell them what they should be doing without actually *telling* them. "Do you think we should draw a blood culture now?" Or, "Do you think we should call your senior resident about this?" Of course, what they *mean* is, "We *should* draw a blood culture now. We *should* page your senior resident about this," but framing it as a question allows us as the doctors, we who are supposedly issuing the orders, to save face.

Another way that nurses deal with inexperienced doctors is just to bypass them altogether. If there's anything truly menial that needs to be done by an MD (filling out a requisition slip, signing off on something inconsequential), they will page the intern, but otherwise, the nurses will skip right over us and go to the senior resident with their question or concern. Sometimes I actually don't mind this—it *does* save time, because at this point, almost any *real* question nurses pose I would have to turn around and relay to my senior resident anyway. This saves me the trouble of having to play this elaborate game of telephone, since running down the senior, clarifying the question, and then finding the nurse again can sometimes take upward of an hour. But then again, there is something galling about my value on the team being so completely discounted.

The third way that nurses deal with interns is by yelling at them. I am currently becoming intimately acquainted with this approach.

Earlier that day on rounds, we decided (that is to say, my seniors and the attending on service decided, and I wrote it down) that one of my patients required a blood transfusion. The patient is a two-month-old boy with a host of ill-defined medical problems, and over the past week or so in the hospital, his blood count has been steadily declining, possibly related to disease, but also probably due to the fact that we are drawing two or three vials of blood from him per day in an attempt to find a diagnosis. Having never ordered a blood transfusion for a baby before, I wasn't really sure how *much* blood to order, but reasoned that whatever volume we were going to eventually infuse, I should probably order the smallest possible amount. I am aware that blood comes packaged from the blood bank in "units," which are the little plastic bags that you see at the blood bank, after the needle but before the cookies and juice. This baby is only about 9 pounds, so I figure I would order as little as I could to avoid waste. Therefore, I put in an order for one unit, or approximately 250 cubic centimeters (ccs), of packed red blood cells.

"Are you *kidding* me?" Cindy, a senior nurse on the floor is asking me, as if she expects me to actually answer in the affirmative, *Yes, I was just kidding. April Fool's!* "One whole *unit* of packed reds? For this little baby? *Look* at this thing!" She holds up the bag of blood and waves it in front of my nose. "It's as big as he is!"

"Um..." This is not going well. I try to think of what I should say. Should I explain? Defend myself? Yell back? All of this is making me dizzy. "See, the thing is...when I...that...if you..." What the hell was I trying to say? *Think, woman, think!* I begin again. "I didn't think that I could order anything *less* than a unit from the blood bank. I figured when the blood came up, we would give him as much as he needed for his transfusion, but I never intended that he should get the *whole thing.*" It occurs to me then that while I never intended to transfuse the whole bag, I'm not actually sure how much exactly I *had* wanted my patient to get. A fifth of the bag? One hundred ccs? One point twenty-one gigawatts?

"*Look* at this! And now we're going to have to waste this *whole unit* of blood! Imagine if we *had* tried to give this whole unit! We could have gotten fired! The kid could have *died*! It would have been in all the papers!" Cindy is on a roll now, really fired up; there is clearly no stopping her. Given a little more time, she could probably extend this story to a dramatic and satisfying end with me being led away in handcuffs, a sweatshirt draped over my bowed head. QUACK DOC ARRESTED FOR IDIOCY, the banner headline in the *New York Post* would read, right next to a picture of last night's Mega Millions winner, grinning and holding a sheaf of hundred-dollar bills in front of him like a fan.

I try once again to explain that I had not been intending to actually transfuse the *whole* unit, that this is not quite a medical error, more of a procedural misunderstanding on my part with respect to how the blood bank ordering system works—when my senior resident steps in. "Cindy, I've got this. How long has this blood been out?"

She calms down instantly upon seeing him, and I think, a little sulkily, that nurses like the male residents better, treat them differently. *They love the guys, defer to them more automatically; they can have that whole flirty 1950s doctor-nurse thing going on. Women don't get the same kind of response.* "About forty-five minutes," she replies sweetly, reporting the amount of time the unit of blood has been sitting at room temperature, out of refrigeration.

"Great, so we still have more than three hours. Send the unit back down to the blood bank and have them draw off forty ccs. They can still save the rest, we didn't use any, and it'll still be good by the time it gets back down to them." He puts his hand on my shoulder. "Let's go back to the team room."

In the team room, a workstation where the junior residents spend most of their time occupied with all manner of computerized scut, he turns to face me and puts a hand on my shoulder. "You obviously didn't know this, but usually, the calculation for the volume of packed red blood cells to transfuse is ten to fifteen ccs per kilogram. Your patient weighs four kilos, so..."

"He should get forty ccs of blood," I finish, recalling what he just told the nurse outside. "But *can* you just order forty ccs of blood from the blood bank? I thought it was stored in those big unit bags."

"It is, and usually for adults, they order one unit, two units, whatever. For kids, though, they'll draw off whatever volume we need and stick it in a smaller bag or, for the *really* little kids, into syringes." He smiles, not quite wanting to convey that I didn't make a mistake, but also not wanting to make me feel worse than I clearly already do. "So now you know," he ends simply.

I breathe out deeply. "Now I know." Then, feeling as though I have let him down, I say, "Sorry."

"Come on," he says. And then he tells me something that sticks with me for the rest of my training. "You're not *supposed* to know everything yet. If you did, what would be the point of residency?" Reassuringly, he claps me on the shoulder twice and adds, "You're doing fine," before walking away, off to bail the next green July intern out from yet another crisis.

It occurs to me then what a chaotic place the hospital is in July. There is the everyday chaos, of course—that is unavoidable—but there's also the chaos of having people newly promoted to all new roles, feeling them out and learning what they're supposed to do on the job, while real patients, no less sick than they were on June 30, stand by for us to sort things out. I am new in my role, having been a medical student just a few weeks ago, but so is almost everyone else. My senior resident is learning how to lead and supervise, giving enough support without micromanaging and getting swamped in the minutiae of the juniors. The fellows on the wards are new too, having gained induction into their subspecialty trades just days after graduating from residency themselves, and some of the attendings are also inexperienced, either fresh graduates or new hires, not yet sure of their roles within the hierarchy. The only people who *aren't* new, really, are the nurses, and I understand now why I've been told that the more senior nurses with the most pull try to arrange their vacation time for at least part of the month of July so as to avoid the worst of this transition period. *Remind me never to get admitted to the hospital in July,* I tell myself with a shudder, unaware that two years from now, I will be delivering my first child at this very hospital on July 22.

Later that afternoon, I walk up to Cindy, who is sitting at the nursing station. She has calmed down. When she turns around to look at me, I can tell that in her own prickly way, she's sorry about the scene we had earlier. Wordlessly, I hand her a handful of strawberry-flavored Laffy Taffy, which I picked up at the hospital gift shop in the lobby.

She looks down at the candy. "What's all this about?"

I shrug. "I just figured that it must be hard for nurses in July. All us new kids running around, screwing things up. Just give me a few more days to get up to speed. Then, you know, I'll be *awesome* at this job." We both laugh at the lie, unwrap the taffy, and dive in.

* * *

There is one piece of equipment you get when you start your third year of medical school, one thing that sets you apart from first- and second-year medical students, and that thing is a pager. We had to pay for them out of our own pockets, and they didn't sport any of the more advanced features that the residents' pagers had, like the ability to send text messages—but still, what could be more doctor-y than having a *pager* on your belt? We spent the entire first half of the year glowing about our new toys, fussily checking them, choosing which ring tone we wanted (was a series of chirps more professional, or the single, piercing beep?) and trying not to squeal with glee whenever someone actually paged us. "Oh, who's paging me *now?*" we'd groan, as though we got paged *all the time* instead of maybe twice a week, tops, mimicking the harassed, *oh lord what now* annoyance we learned from shadowing our overworked residents, all the while inwardly rejoicing about how important it made us seem.

But two years later, by the end of my first week

as an intern, I am just about ready to throw my pager out the window. A *high* window. Overlooking a trash compactor. Filled with highly corrosive acid. How could I have ever thought that it was cool to get paged? How could I ever have *enjoyed* carrying a pager? How could I have ever *not* been aggravated to tears by the sound of that beeping and *beeping* and BEEPING and *OH MY GOD WHY WON'T YOU EVER STOP BEEPING?* Years later, long after residency, the sound of a pager will still trigger a Pavlovian response in me, a combination of dread, an uptick in pulse, and an involuntary reaching toward my right hip where, once, my pager was welded.

It is my first night on overnight call early in July, and the entire evening has been a flurry of admissions, one after the other, from the Emergency Room. My pager is, of course, going off constantly, nurses calling from one ward, then the next, and my legs are trembling and jellylike from running up and down the stairwell. Much later in the year, out of curiosity, I will strap on a pedometer at the start of one twenty-four-hour call period and log the distance I have traveled during my shift. By the following morning, I will have logged 8.3 miles just from running between wards.

My next admission has just hit the floor, a five-week-old baby admitted to rule out sepsis. "Rule out sepsis" admissions are the bread and butter of the inpatient pediatrics ward—basically surveillance and observation admissions for any baby less than two months old who comes in with a fever greater than 100.4°F. We do not admit all children with fevers—in older children, we basically expect them—but in very young babies, who haven't had their first set of vaccinations, a fever can indicate more significant systemic infections, like meningitis contracted near or at the time of birth, which could have grave consequences if not treated promptly and correctly. All babies presenting for a rule-out-sepsis workup have blood, urine, and cerebrospinal fluid drawn in the Emergency Room and sent for culture (the cerebrospinal fluid draw is conceptually the most distressing for parents, as it involves a spinal tap), and are administered IV antibiotics for at least forty-eight hours, until the results of these cultures come back, usually negative. Most nights on call, a resident can expect at least one rule-out-sepsis admission, and by the spring, most residents are able to do these admissions in their sleep. I even did a few as a medical student, so when my senior resident sends me in with the breezy instructions, "It's just a rule-out sepsis, you know what to do, right? Call me if you need anything," I am happy to be entrusted with this level of autonomy and rush to comply.

I walk into the patient's room shortly after he and his mother arrive on the floor from the ER at 4:30 a.m. It is a double room, and the other patient is a toddler, whose mother is sleeping in a fold-out chair next to her crib and snoring lightly. The baby admitted to rule out sepsis, *my* patient, is lying in his own crib, still awake and wrapped in a plush blue fleece, looking rosy and cherubic and lovely. His mother, appearing a little more tired, looks up and says hello. She is attractive and in her midthirties, casually but elegantly dressed despite her recent ordeal in the ER, and looks every bit the stereotype of the Upper West Side alphamom. On one hand, this is a relief—I was worried that I would have to conduct my history and physical exam in Spanish, which in Washington Heights we are often called upon to do, though at this hour of the morning and with my rudimentary language skills, it was not a challenge that I relished. But on the other hand, these alphamoms always make me slightly nervous, though whether this nervousness stems from their demeanor or my own insecurities I can't say.

"Hi, my name is Michelle Au, I'm one of the Pediatric residents on the floor. I know you've been through a lot already, and I'm going to make sure that you and"—quick flick of the eye to the baby's chart—"Aiden can get some rest tonight, but to be complete, I'm going to just reconfirm some things about his medical history and do a quick physical exam, just so we can best take care of him while he's here."

"I hope you don't take this the wrong way," Aiden's mother interjects, "but how long have you been doing this?"

"Doing what?" I don't quite understand the question.

"How long have you been a doctor?" she clarifies. And there it is, the question that I've been dreading all week.

I weigh my various options before answering, but aside from flat-out lying, I see no way around this. "I started my internship on Monday."

"So four days, then." She purses her lips. "I'm sorry, I'd just really rather my son be followed by a more senior doctor."

I flush, embarrassed. "He will be," I assure her, "I work as part of a team. The entire team will round on Aiden tomorrow morning, and an attending physician oversees all the patients on the team, in addition to a senior Pediatrics resident. We all work together."

"Well then, I'll wait for the attending to come in later in the morning," the mother answers. She hardens her mouth into a line, seeing that I am somewhat at a loss for words. "Look, I'm not trying to be difficult. I just think that he's been through enough. Did you know that it took them half an hour to get that spinal tap on him downstairs? *Half an hour!* He's three weeks old! He's had enough, and *I've* had enough. I know this is a teaching hospital, but I don't want any more people 'practicing' on my baby tonight. We'll see the attending in the morning."

I try to parry, explaining that there will be no more needles, that the purpose of my interview is purely to round out the history and to conduct a physical exam, and pick up on any details that may have been missed in the chaos of the ER. But she is firm. She will allow my attending to examine her child, and the attending only. *But that's not allowed,* I want to say to her, only the thinnest barrier of restraint keeping my sleep-deprived brain from saying these things out loud, *I'm the one who's supposed to do it. This is a rule-out-sepsis admission, pure low-level scut; what's my senior resident going to say when she finds out I couldn't even get this done?* Finally, after a few more rebuffed advances, I mumble something about talking it over with the senior on call and exit the room, trying to plan my next step.

My first reaction, after the initial embarrassment, is anger. *How dare she pick and choose? This is a teaching hospital! This is how it works! I may be young, but I'm still a doctor! She wants the best of both worlds, the benefit of having her son at an academic medical center while dealing only with the attending like at a private hospital! But when you're admitted to a teaching hospital, you have to play by the rules! If she doesn't want to respect the system, she should really just go somewhere else.*

The problem is, my own self-righteous indignation aside, on a deeper level I actually agree with her. What if he were *my* baby? What if I were sitting in that room after watching some resident struggling to correctly place a 1 1/2-inch needle into my baby's spinal column after repeated attempts? Who *wouldn't* want to see a more senior doctor? Who *wouldn't* see a twenty-four-year-old intern walking in, disheveled and sleep deprived, stray bits of paper poking out of the pockets of her white coat and scrubs, and demand someone better? She *shouldn't* trust me. Even *I* don't trust me. What the hell do *I* know? How presumptuous to think that any parent who knows that their child could potentially be ill, and knows that I have next to no clinical experience, would let me fumble along anyway?

The idea of the bumbling intern doing some Three Stooges routine on a patient isn't entirely accurate—after all, we are almost always supervised, especially while doing procedures, and we are supposed to direct any questions, large or small, up the chain of command, to make sure that mistakes are avoided and that inexperience is compensated for. But at the core, it *is* true. We are not as technically proficient or as experienced as our senior residents or our attendings. How can we be? In the sense that we can only get better after repeated attempts, we *are* "practicing" on our patients. And it's hard for a four-day-old intern already filled with self-doubt to argue with a mother that she does have the requisite experience to take responsibility for her baby's medical care. I don't have to hear her argument. She's preaching to the choir.

In the end, I try again half an hour later, dragging my third-year resident in with me as a human shield. My senior introduces herself warmly, somehow emphasizing her seniority without calling more attention to my lack of the same, and somehow, either with her manner or her words, smoothes things over. She then stands off to the side, not saying another word, and I conduct the history and physical as I would have were she not there, looking to her only occasionally to see if she wants to double-check the patient's lung exam (she does) or the ear exam (she does not). The mom is cordial to us, even thanks us when we leave. As for the issue of seniority or my lack thereof, it does not come up again, and on rounds the following morning my senior merely mentions at the end of my presentation that the mother is "a little high maintenance," and we move on to the next patient, who is on the waiting list for a liver transplant.

I see Aiden only a few more times, and his admission is as smooth as anyone could hope, all his cultures negative, his intravenous antibiotics discontinued after forty-eight hours, and he is discharged back home shortly thereafter. Still, in those forty-eight hours, every time I walk by his room, I feel that same flush of outrage and embarrassment, as well as that same sense of vulnerability and exposure, remembering the night that his mother publicly called me out, and correctly so, as a fraud.

* * *

My civilian friends—all two of them—keep asking me if it feels *different* to finally be a resident rather than a medical student. I would like to say yes, perhaps brandishing a few new war stories or a bloodstained cuff of my lab coat as proof of my machismo, but I have to say, it really doesn't feel different at all. I still don't know what the hell is going on, I still can't write prescriptions (my hospital-provided malpractice insurance doesn't kick in until the end of my second week), and I still don't have my keys to the resident call room. My last night on call, I managed to catch an hour and a half of sleep very early in the morning, but I had to do it propped up on the couch in the back of the patient playroom, which is painted with eerily psychedelic forest murals. Given that I have nowhere else to go, the playroom is actually my secret hideout at night, but I try not to publicize that fact because I'm pretty sure that I'm not really allowed in there. This is probably not the glamorous image the hospital wants to project, that rumpled and vaguely homeless-looking house staff are routinely passed out in the back room, next to the Radio Flyer wagon and Lincoln Logs.

While I am starting my internship, Joe is also starting across town, at Mount Sinai Hospital on the Upper East Side. Though he will be starting his residency in Ophthalmology the following year, as with many specialized fields of medicine (such as dermatology, radiology, or neurosurgery), a preliminary year, or "prelim," is required to give new graduates an appreciation of the scope and depth of general medicine before narrowing down their focus to just one organ.

We are both flush from the whirlwind of our wedding and honeymoon, and excited for ourselves and each other to finally start our residencies—but the reality that we both understand is that for the first four years of our marriage, we will be spending significantly more time at the hospital than we will with each other. As if to drive this point home, the first two weeks of Joe's internship will be spent on the general medicine wards doing "night float," meaning that he will be working nights, and *only* nights, for fourteen days straight.

Night float forces you to adopt an unnatural, nocturnal lifestyle. Most residents on night float come home from work in the mornings, sleep during the day, and then return to work later that evening. Sleeping during the day can obviously be an issue, especially living as we do, in an apartment with upstairs neighbors in the midst of renovations (from

137

the sound of things, they are actively drilling into every square inch of wall—perhaps they are fitness buffs building their own pegboard?) and in that peri-student state of partially furnished housing, with no blinds on our windows. There is that constant woozy jetlagged feeling, to which one of course adjusts by the end of two weeks, just in time for the end of the tour of overnight duty, requiring a re-acclimation to a more traditional diurnal rhythm.

Probably the most difficult thing during any prolonged period of working nights, however, is the complete disconnect from the daylight world. You are at work when everyone else is off, you are off when everyone else is at work. Though Joe and I technically live in the same home, we are separated as though we reside in alternate dimensions. All we have as proof that the other still exists is the trace residue that not very tidy people leave during the ordinary course of living—a pair of dirty socks near the doorway, a plate with crumbs on the counter, a rumpled bed that still holds the imprint of a sleeper not long vacated. We leave notes for each other, occasionally talk on the phone when the one who's working is less busy, but otherwise, we live in opposite though parallel universes.

Toward the end of the first week, however, we come upon a temporizing measure. It is not a "date night" (since Joe is working nights) and it's not breakfast together (since I leave for work at 5:00 a.m.), but still, it's *something*. Most days, around the time that I am heading home, Joe is leaving the house to head into work, and with some coordination, we can bump into each other going in opposite directions and manage to talk face to face for about five minutes. This point of intersection happens to be on the street—at the corner of 23rd Street and Park Avenue, near the entrance to the uptown number six train—but we will exploit whatever overlap in our schedules we can.

We cut a strange sight—two blue scrub–clad adults, holding what looks like a medical consultation at the top of the stairs as the throngs of commuters ebb and flow around us, but we hardly notice. We try to pack into these five minutes a day as much as we can, hastily exchanging necessary household information (the dog threw up today, the lightbulb over the sink blew out), helpful tips (I saved you half of my sandwich from lunch, it's in the fridge if you want it), and amusing updates about patients and coresidents from our respective shifts at work. Toward the end of our daily five-minute subway summit, we inevitably devolve to a spate of in-jokes and endearments, talking faster and faster, voices overlapping, before we send each other off to go our separate ways.

"Man," I remarked one evening standing outside the subway station, looking at my watch and realizing that, once again, our daily time together had run out. "How do people do this? I've seen you for maybe a total of twenty minutes this entire week. And we just started residency, there's still four years of this left, at least. This blows."

"Yeah," Joe agreed, removing a fare card from his wallet and preparing to descend into the station. "It blows. But that's what we signed up for, I guess." And before I can figure out whether this pronouncement makes me feel inspired or just depressed, he's already gone, swallowed up by the sepulchral gloom of the subway station.

Justin

It's 3:00 a.m., and I am walking the halls of the hospital prowling for morphine.

I am the resident on call for the Pediatric Oncology service, and on the floor tonight I have a patient who is dying. He's a teenage boy named Justin who has been dying for weeks now with end-stage Ewing's sarcoma, which has spread to almost all of his vital organs, and in the past few days he has been requiring higher and higher doses of medication for pain. A few days ago, the Pediatric Pain service placed Justin on a continuous morphine infusion with additional doses that could be self-administered, in the effort to allow his passing to be as comfortable and painless as possible for him and his family.

The morphine has helped, and made him sleepy as well, though not sleepy enough to stop him from groggily turning to his parents a few times an hour to tell them, "I'm dying. I'm scared." It is heartbreaking, and unnerving as well, to watch someone die who *knows* he's dying and who is aware enough to really understand what that means. I found myself walking by Justin's room a couple of times earlier in the night, just to peek in the window, feeling macabre, and not really sure if I was checking for something specific or if it's just to comfort myself that he's still there. Every time I looked in, he was sleeping, vital signs steady on the screen overhead, his thumb resting lightly on the dosage button of the patient-controlled analgesia machine.

So when Justin's nurse came into the doctor's workroom just before 2:00 a.m. and sat down with a sigh, I got a little worried. "The satellite pharmacy just called me," she said. Satellite pharmacies are off-shoots of the central pharmacy that supply specific areas of the hospital—the operating rooms, the intensive care units, the emergency rooms. This particular satellite pharmacy that Justin's nurse was referring to supplies the general medical wards of the Children's Hospital.

"And?"

"And they're out of morphine."

"The satellite pharmacy is out of morphine," I repeated, just to try to process what she was saying. If I were a normal person, I would have been home now, in bed. Perhaps I would have been having that anxiety dream that I always have wherein I have to take the final exam for a high school math class I didn't even know I had registered for. But I would have been sleeping at least. "Do we have enough for him?"

"I don't think so. Not for the whole night. We only have"—I could see her eyes getting hazy as she did the calculations—"about two hundred milligrams left."

"I see. And what's the problem? Why can't they just get some more? They're the *pharmacy*."

"They said that Central Pharmacy is closed until eight a.m.," the nurse told me. "It's locked up, and they don't have access until the morning. All they have is what's in the satellite pharmacy, and we already used up all the morphine that they have."

"How much morphine is he using per hour at this point?" The nurse went to get Justin's chart, and we pored over it. "Let's see...basal dose...he got four demand doses...add those..." I tapped the figures into the calculator on a chain I always have hanging around my neck, like a nerdy version of Flavor Flav's giant clock. "Wait, is that right? *That's* how much he's using? That's a *crazy* amount of morphine. He's still *breathing* on all that?"

"Breathing, talking," the nurse confirmed. "It helps him sleep, though."

"So at this current rate, he's going to run out of morphine at about"—I did the calculations quickly— "six a.m."

"Right."

"And Central Pharmacy doesn't open until eight a.m."

"Right."

"So where are we going to find more morphine?"

"That's why I came to find you."

"Ah. I've finally caught up."

And that is why, at 3:00 a.m., I am walking the halls, trying to find someone to help me score some morphine for my patient. I need enough to bridge the gap between six and about nine (figuring in some extra time for the pharmacy to actually open and compound the drug), and I am acutely aware of the clock ticking, the supply that we have running out.

The kid, I think, *is dying.* He doesn't need to be in any more pain than he is already experiencing, and he certainly doesn't need to go into withdrawal. I think back to last week—before Justin was started on his morphine infusion, the way he had been wild, screaming and crying—and am aware that, to some degree, I am also trying to spare his parents and caregivers the pain of having to watch him suffer. Certainly, there are other drugs that I could give him to tide him over after the morphine runs out, but at the high doses he is receiving and with my uncertain understanding of palliative care and the pharmacokinetics of the drugs, I am hesitant to fiddle with the Pain Management team's recommendations, especially since the regimen they have him on seems to be working well. I just need to find the kid enough morphine to get him through the night.

I stop by the general medicine ward, the cardiac ward, and even call down to the Emergency Room, with no luck. Given that the satellite pharmacy is supplying the entire Children's Hospital, the other wards don't have any supply that those of us on the oncology ward don't have access to as well. It is now past 4:00 a.m. I walk by Justin's room again. He is sleeping soundly, his parents rumpled and snoring on the pull-out bed in the corner. The nurse is in his room, changing the bag on the patient-controlled analgesia machine. She points to the morphine and holds up one finger, indicating that there is only one infusion bag remaining in our supply and that she is hanging it now. I nod that I understand.

Finally, in desperation, I head up to the Pediatric ICU. They have a good number of postsurgical patients, a few who are on morphine drips themselves.

So I know they at least have a stock of the medication on the floor. The question is whether they have enough to spare. I look for a sympathetic-looking nurse (I don't really know what such a nurse would look like, but one looks like a good bet, as she is young and does not appear to be polishing her knife collection) and approach her.

"Hi. I'm Michelle, one of the residents covering the Oncology service down on five."

"Hey, Michelle. What are you doing visiting us up here?"

"I need to ask a favor." And I explain the situation, stressing that the medication is running at an extremely high dose, but that Justin has end-stage metastatic cancer and this is a palliative care situation, for a patient who will be dying in a matter of days, not weeks. "The pain regimen he's on now is working for him, and I really don't want to screw around with that, you know? I mean, you should have seen him before we started the drip. It was..." I think back again on Justin's panicky gasps for air, his guttural moans of pain, with his parents weeping next to him all the while. "It was just not good," I conclude.

"Wow, poor kid," says the nurse, who is indeed sympathetic. "Let me see if we can help you out. What was his name again?" I tell her. "Well, let's just see what we have here." She walks over to the Pyxis, a squat gray machine with many locked drawers, kind of a bank ATM for controlled substances. She enters her access code and finds the patient on the list of the hospital census. "A morphine PCA, you said?"

"Morphine," I confirm.

"We have patients on morphine PCAs up here right now," she says cheerfully, punching in the appropriate information, "but most of them are pretty little, and the doses they're on are pretty small, so I think we have some extra." With a pop, one of the drawers opens and the nurse removes a few bottles from the shelves within. "Do you think this will be enough for the next few hours?" She has handed me about 400 mg of morphine. More narcotics than I have ever handled in my entire life. I suddenly start to feel very nervous.

I am not quite sure what to do with my hands, with the bottles. Do I hold them gingerly out in front of me, or will everyone see what I'm carrying and get suspicious? Or would putting them in my pocket look even more suspicious? After thanking her again I take my leave, taking care not to walk too fast, lest I seem, I don't know, too *eager* to abscond with my gigantic fistfuls of morphine.

In the elevator on my way back down to the oncology ward, I look at the sheer quantity of narcotic in my hands with a kind of wonder. I still can't believe she just handed this to me. *How could she trust me? I could have been lying. I could be a drug addict. I could have made up that whole sob story about the dying kid. I could be leaving the building to sell this stuff on the street right now.* And then a different thought occurred to me. *What if a real junkie sees me? What if he sees that I'm carting around enough morphine to kill a horse, and decides to jam a shiv between my ribs and steal the whole stash?* Looking around furtively, I decide to put the medication in my pockets after all.

Back on the oncology ward, I find Justin's nurse and gratefully surrender the morphine to her. "Don't ask me how I got this," I say before she can open her mouth, "it involved prostitution." Relieved to be absolved of the responsibility of guarding the narcotics, I scurry back to the doctors' lounge to pick up my notes so that I can make some predawn rounds on the rest of the patients on the floor. It is now almost 5:00 a.m.

Most nights on call, residents occupy themselves with crisis management, or "putting out fires," as we somewhat irreverently refer to the process of keeping all our patients alive until everyone arrives back for work in the morning. The day team usually does their part by "tucking in" their patients before they leave work for the day, clearing out all miscellaneous tasks, and making sure that each patient is taken care of so far as can be anticipated for the night, thereby keeping nocturnal scut to a minimum. Usually, despite these efforts, nights pass in a low-grade frenzy of activity anyway. Drawing late-night blood cultures on patients with fevers, admitting patients from the Emergency Room, ordering portable chest X-rays and medications for patients who suddenly decide that breathing is a lot harder than it sounds. Or some nights, like tonight, the main task at hand is just to ensure that your patient and his family are able to sleep through the night.

Justin passed away comfortably a few days later, his parents by his side. He was seventeen years old.

Emergency

The unfortunate thing about medical training, the thing that nobody tells you, is that the exact things for which you are valued in your medical school application—altruism, patience, well-rounded interests with numerous extracurricular hobbies, an all-around compassion for humanity—are the exact things that are beaten out of you during the years it takes you to become a doctor. And nowhere is this more true for me than during my rotations in the Pediatric Emergency Room.

I hate working in the Pediatric Emergency Room.

The Emergency Room is the Wild Wild West of the hospital, the unsheltered front line of medicine, where any and all patients can stumble in and, if they don't mind the ten-hour wait time, eventually even be seen by a doctor. Some medical people love this environment, thriving on the unpredictability, the chaos, the excitement of receiving patients off the street, off the backs of squealing ambulances, unlabeled and undiagnosed, having to decide who is sick enough to stay and who should go home. During the 2008 election, there was a great deal of discussion about the number of Americans without health insurance who, lacking other options, used the Emergency Department as their primary care facility. And maybe some don't mind that either, dealing with patients who show up to the ER because they need a prescription refilled or because they need new glasses. But in my experience, no matter how nice they are, most doctors I've met do not find this a good use of Emergency Room manpower or resources.

You have to first understand what it's like to work in a busy ER. Picture one of those railroad stations in Calcutta, with tense, sweaty bodies pressed together, stomach to back, all angry and rushed and surging for the trains, which are already filled to capacity and have passengers and luggage hanging off the tops and out the sides. Throw in a couple of barn animals, maybe the sound of an air raid siren blaring overhead. Add on the chorus of a half dozen infants with diarrhea crying in dissonant harmony. Then pretend that a nurse, one of your attendings, and an extremely irate parent are all talking to you simultaneously about three separate things while your pager is going off. All while you're getting sprayed by a fire hose. Now you're getting close.

Though theoretically I would have thought that working the ER would be somehow gratifying—making diagnoses from scratch, occasional made-for-TV excitement, giving back to the community by serving the underserved—overall I find that my time in the ER is turning me into a person that I don't want to be. I start to always feel rushed, even when I'm not at work, a panicky feeling that makes me check my watch compulsively and feel that the normal pace of life outside the hospital is much too slow to be tolerated. Ordering coffee at one of the mobile sidewalk carts near the hospital, I will watch them spoon in the sugar and add the cream, silently seething the entire thirty seconds while in my head I am screaming, OH MY GOD, JUST POUR IT FASTER, MAN.

Waiting on line for the bathroom, actually listening at the door for the sounds of events transpiring inside, I bounce back and forth, not with any sort of excretory urgency but because I am just *enraged*, wondering, WHY THE HELL ARE YOU TAKING SO LONG, WHAT, DID YOU *DIE* IN THERE? Once I got stuck in a stairwell behind a woman who, aside from being rather large, was in no particular hurry to get to her office, and I had to really exert extreme control to prevent myself from sighing audibly, pushing her to one side, and running up those steps two at a time. WALK FASTER, WOMAN, YOU WORK IN A HOSPITAL.

In addition to superimposing this sense of imperturbable hurry into everything I have to do, I also start to become something of a misanthrope. Pediatricians by nature are a fuzzy bunch, prone to hugging patients and wearing cutesy charms in the holes of their Crocs, but I see a lot of aggrieved looks and rolling eyes pass between residents while working in the Emergency Room. When I take care of a three-year-old boy whose parents called an ambulance (*an ambulance!*) because, having been allowed to eat a diet solely consisting of birthday cake and Halloween candy for the past twenty-four hours, the kid understandably developed a stomachache, I find it difficult not to get annoyed and sarcastic with his parents about their judgment. Which is to say that, while I rarely say anything overt, I walk out of a good number of examination rooms cracking my knuckles and muttering to myself, *What is wrong with these people?*

One night, or rather, early one morning, I bring a mother and her two-year-old into one of the exam rooms and lead off with my standard question: "So, what brings you to the Emergency Room today?"

The mother responds, "She had a nosebleed." After some questioning, I determine that the nosebleed actually happened four days ago and stopped on its own after five minutes, with no further episodes since. Perhaps lacking anything further to say, the mother offers, "Here, look, some of it got on the blanket." She takes a flowered pink security blanket out of her purse, where sure enough, a small dot of dried blood, smaller than my pinkie nail, is visible. The child, happy, rambunctious, definitely not bleeding to death, sits in the corner and starts gnawing at the bulb of the blood pressure cuff.

I pause for a long time, blinking. And then I say, very slowly, "So *that's* the reason you brought your child to the Emergency Room at four a.m. on a Sunday?"

The Emergency Room is turning me into kind of an asshole.

To be fair, the reason we have developed such short fuses for these nonemergencies is because, at this hospital, there is no shortage of *real* emergencies in the Pediatric ER. For every patient who has been dragged in by his parents for sneezing twice and not quite having the appetite to finish his Whopper Jr., we have patients who are septic, patients on respirators, patients who have been stabbed on their way home from school, and unstable patients with complex congenital heart malformations. When you have just taken care of a cancer patient with no immune defenses left after chemotherapy who appears to not only be growing gram-negative bacteria in his blood but also has a platelet count so low that at any moment he could start spontaneously bleeding into his brain, suddenly your level of patience for dealing with a patient who has been sent in from school for toenail fungus becomes very low. It's not that as doctors, we don't like to deal with otherwise well patients, or that we're not used to seeing patients for maintenance issues like immunizations or summer-camp physicals. But having to deal with these issues in the Emergency Room feels like watering flowers in a war zone: *this is neither the time nor the place.*

One of my coresidents summed up this sentiment best during the end of one particularly grueling shift, with the line of patients waiting to be seen spilling out of the waiting room into the hospital atrium, rows of colored patient charts blooming from every rack like hardy wildflowers after a rain on the prairie. "Man," he said bitterly, hurriedly scratching out a prescription for asthma medication while simultaneously checking an X-ray on the computer system, "if you ain't dying tonight, stay the hell out of the ER."

* * *

The thing about the ER is that it can be a little like working in a casino. It doesn't matter what the clock says—and there are no windows to give you any sense of time passing—your task is always the same. Pick up a chart, see a patient. Pick up a chart, see a patient. Not sure what to do next? Why not try picking up a chart and seeing a patient? Repeat one million times (give or take) until your shift ends, or you die, whichever comes first. In the Pediatric Emergency Room, however, there does seem to be some sort of a biorhythm to the day, with types of patients and activities falling into distinct chunks over the twenty-four-hour cycle. And, having worked all hours in the Pediatric ER at Columbia, I find myself breaking up the day not into shifts, but into case types.

8:00 a.m.—3:00 p.m.: All Comers

Your standard mix of emergency and not-so-emergency patients. Think of the show *ER*, except with much-less-attractive people. Though this is not necessarily the busiest time of day in the Emergency Room, it is often the best staffed, with anywhere from four to six medical students milling around at all times, doing that excruciating med-student dance of trying to be as helpful and eager yet as unobtrusive as possible, occasionally failing on all counts. Therefore, even with few patients in the Emergency Room during the mornings, it always feels crowded. Additionally, daylight business hours are also the most common time of day to receive patients like this:

MICHELLE: Good morning, I'm Dr. Au, one of the Pediatrics residents working in the Emergency Room. So, what brings you to the ER today?

EIGHTEEN-YEAR-OLD GIRL: I came to the ER because I don't know why I can't get pregnant.

MICHELLE: *(A little surprised)* Wait, you *want* to get pregnant?

EIGHTEEN-YEAR-OLD GIRL: Yeah.

MICHELLE: And you're upset because you're not.

EIGHTEEN-YEAR-OLD GIRL: Yeah, me and my boyfriend been trying to get a baby [*sic*] for six months, but it hasn't been working.

MICHELLE: And you're sure that *you* want to get pregnant too, not that your boyfriend is pressuring you or...

EIGHTEEN-YEAR-OLD GIRL: No, no, we *both* want to have kids. But I want to make sure there's not something wrong with me because it's not working so far.

MICHELLE: You know, this is really more of an issue for your regular medical doctor.

EIGHTEEN-YEAR-OLD GIRL: Yeah, but this is *important.*

MICHELLE: Well, there isn't much in the Emergency Room that we can do for that, but since it's not so busy in here now, I'll tell you what. I'll do a routine exam and maybe we can send some simple cultures and blood tests, just so that when you *do* make an appointment with your regular doctor, she can have something to start with. But an infertility workup, if that's really what you have, isn't something that's done in the ER.

EIGHTEEN-YEAR-OLD GIRL: *(Impatiently)* Is this going to take a long time? The exam and the tests?

MICHELLE: A little while, why?

EIGHTEEN-YEAR-OLD GIRL: I have to go. I have an appointment in half an hour.

MICHELLE: Where? With whom?

EIGHTEEN-YEAR-OLD GIRL: With my gynecologist.

(Michelle hurls self in front of truck.)

3:00 p.m.–6:00 p.m.: The After-School Melee

For obvious reasons, this is a time when we see a lot of teenage trauma, where kids who are walking home from school—on their way to church choir practice, or en route to their volunteer jobs at the orphanage, no doubt—get jumped. Most of the injuries are not serious, mostly of the bruises and scrapes variety, and the story is almost always the same. "I didn't *know* them, I wasn't doing *anything*, just these five guys came out of nowhere and started beating on me!" Not that all these patients are boys. I've had more than a few girls coming in after getting mauled by what sounds like some roving all-girl gang, like something out of *Faster, Pussycat! Kill! Kill!*

6:00 p.m.–11:00 p.m.: The After-Dinner Specials

One of the busiest stretches, and also a peak time for people to bring their children into the ER for seemingly no good reason whatsoever. "Hey kids, we've all had dinner, we're all still awake, what you say we take a big family trip down to the Emergency Room and check out what's playing on that little TV they have out in the waiting room?" *"Yeah! Great idea, Dad!"* In my more sympathetic moments, I realize that this is in part because many parents are off in the evenings, and those without good access to primary care often have to resort to visiting the ER during nonwork hours when they know they can be seen without an appointment, regardless of insurance or immigration status. And yet, I wonder if those people who drag an entire brood of healthy children into the

ER for some spurious reason realize that if you're not sick when you come to the germ-laden ER, you certainly will be when you leave.

11:00 p.m.–2:00 a.m.: Baby Mama Trauma Drama

Particularly when the weather starts to get warmer and people start to get a little more rambunctious, almost every chart that lands in the box in this time frame seems to be some sort of trauma. Laceration repairs, car accidents, and my personal favorite, Kids Who Fall Off Things. Some nights in the spring and summer, it feels like every single kid in Washington Heights under the age of three has decided to climb up on and subsequently fall off of something high. Fell down the stairs, fell off the bed, fell off the bed at the top of the stairs. Which teaches me perhaps the most important lesson about parenthood: *keep your kids strapped down to the floor with gaffer's tape at all times.* Interlaced with almost all of these cases is the omnipresent healthy suspicion of child abuse, so these interviews always take a little longer, getting the stories straight from multiple people if necessary, talking to the child (if he or she can talk), examining him or her for old bruises or scars. Though, honestly, if the story was reasonable and all parties behaving appropriately, would I *really* be able to pick out a child abuser from any other parent whose kid fell off the top of the TV stand? One would hope, but it's impossible to say for sure.

2:00 a.m.–6:00 a.m.: The Autotriage Zone

All bets are off during flu season, but the rest of the

year, the wee hours signal a relatively quiet stretch of the night. Basically, the time of day weeds out all the actual healthy patients (which in the Peds ER, feels like about 75 percent of the patients we usually see) and those kids who actually *do* make it in to see us, who are usually legitimately sick. Unfortunately, it's kind of hard to evaluate these kids sometimes, because when the parents tell you at 4:00 a.m. that the kid is "acting sleepy," you can't tell if he's septic or just normal. Sleepy? Join the club, kid.

6:00 a.m.–8:00 a.m.: The End-of-Shift Gold Rush

They're somewhat sicker than the After-Dinner Specials but healthier than the kids who come in during the Autotriage Zone. Maybe their parents want to squeeze in a quick visit to the ER before work, or they have a fetish about coming to the ER in their pajamas. Equally likely, they're the frequent flyer/chronically ill patients who know enough of what to do for their kids overnight but also know enough about the system that they realize the shortest waits in the ER come during this time. (Helpful hint: Want to work through the ER in less than three hours? Come in at 6:45 a.m.! Mention my name and get a free rectal exam!) Unfortunately, this is also the point of lowest motivation for overnight ER staff. *Couldn't you have waited another fifteen minutes before getting sick, until* after *my shift ended?*

I will say it again: the ER has the strong potential to bring out your inner asshole.

So there are some subtle changes over the twenty-four-hour cycle that, to the experienced eye, can give some clue as to what time of day it is, but otherwise, days and nights in the ER are all pretty much the same, a constant stream of low-grade urgencies punctuated by the occasional heart-stopping emergency. In fact, the only event that allows me to reliably tell time in the ER is the 3:00 a.m. sandwich drop, wherein a café across the street, just prior to receiving their bakery-fresh goods for the morning, drops off heaping mounds of day-olds for the patients and staff of the Peds ER to pick through. Walk through the Peds ER at three thirty in the morning and you will find leftover yogurt cups lined with soggy scrims of granola, see patients attacking chicken salad wraps, and watch ward clerks turn away from their work stations to deal with a mouthful of cheese danish. "Try the turkey sandwich," the attending urges a floridly tattooed teenager with the air of insider knowledge, "the bread is really good." At these times, the ER feels like it could be anyplace where unlikely company is trapped together for an interminable wait. The DMV, the passport office, an airport terminal after all outgoing flights have been canceled due to a storm.

* * *

I am in an exam room, having a conversation that I feel like I must have with different parents at least once a week.

PARENT: *(Indicating her child)* Yeah, he takes some medicine at home.

157

ME: Which medicine, exactly?

PARENT: I don't know.

ME: OK. What is the medicine for?

PARENT: I don't know. They just gave it to me.

ME: Who's "they"?

PARENT: *(Vaguely)* The people at the place.

ME: Ah. *Them.* How many times a day are you giving it to your child?

PARENT: I don't know. It says on the bottle.

ME: Do you have the bottle with you?

PARENT: No.

ME: And *you* don't remember, even though you've been giving him the medication yourself.

PARENT: *(Indignant)* No, I don't *remember.*

ME: Well, let's try this. What does the medicine look like? Is it a pink liquid? Clear? What color is the bottle? The cap?

PARENT: I don't *know.* I don't *look* at it.

ME: OK. Let me just sum this up. You're at home, giving a medication to your child that you don't know the name of, don't know what symptoms the medication is treating, how often you're giving it, don't know who gave it to you or what the actual medication looks like.

PARENT: Yeah. *(Silence)* It ran out though, so could you write me a refill?

I am trying to figure out how to approach this last stumper when one of my attendings knocks on the door and, without waiting for an answer, pokes her head in. "Sorry," she addresses the patient, apologetically, and then to me, "We're going to need you in the trauma bay." I stand up, excuse myself with the promise that I will be back as soon as I can, and exit the room, walking briskly to the back, where a small crowd is gathering.

"There's a teenager found down, EMS is bringing him in," my attending elaborates, putting on gloves and taking off her white coat in preparation. "We don't know much else yet." I follow suit, putting on gloves myself and walking into the trauma bay, where two nurses are busy untangling tubes and unwrapping packages. We are getting ready for a resuscitation.

"Is it a trauma?" I ask, unclear if we should be preparing blood or paging the surgeons on call. But before anyone can answer, EMS arrives. They are pushing a stretcher carrying a large patient, who surprises me by being a girl. She was apparently found unconscious in the bathtub, where the presumption is that she overdosed on prescription psych medication, some her own, some her mother's. The medics are carrying all the bottles they could find on the scene in a small plastic bag. It is unclear whether the patient was already lying down in the bathtub when she overdosed, but it looks as though she might have fallen as well, as there is a large contusion over the left side of her head, with perhaps an attendant bleed underneath. As we move the backboard with the patient over from one stretcher to the other, it is noted that one of her pupils is "blown"—meaning that it is larger than the other pupil, indicating possible herniation of the brain—and that she is no longer breathing.

Resuscitation is always described in the books as a linear process, with handy color-coded flow charts, one intervention pointing neatly to the next. But in reality, everything seems like it is happening at once. I am on one hand trying (and failing) to get vascular access, an attending is on the other arm attempting the same. Nurses are crawling under and in between bodies, positioning monitors, placing defibrillation pads, drawing up medications. Blood is being drawn, tubes of deep maroon passing back and forth over the patient's stripped body and being sent off to the lab stat for analysis. One of the pediatric anesthesiology fellows magically appears and intubates the patient, wincing in disgust when a spray of pink froth issues forth from the tube. "Suction!" he yells, passing the soft suction catheter he is handed down the tube and clearing it as much as he can before hooking it up to the oxygen supply and ventilating the patient by hand. "We have some pulmonary edema here," meaning fluid backing up into the lungs, possibly as a result of cardiac failure. A repeat exam of the patient's eyes now finds both pupils blown. In medicine, particularly in critical care, we talk about patients "circling the drain," meaning patients with a poor prognosis and not getting better, incrementally inching toward death. But this patient is not just circling the drain. She is halfway down it.

Rapidly, the decision is made that the patient needs to be stabilized and sent off for a CT scan to the head to evaluate for herniation of the brain, most likely secondary to bleeding resulting from head trauma, and will be transported straight to the ICU from there. About five people go with the patient for transport, including the anesthesiologist, the emergency attending, a neurosurgical resident, and two nurses. As they clatter down the hall, monitors beeping, support equipment draped over the edge of the stretcher, clogs and sneakers squeaking, they look like a single organism, moving in coordination and somehow insectile. The patient's mother has also shown up in the meantime, and is giving a medical history to another one of the emergency staff, who is writing everything down on a sticky label printed with the patient's name. The mother is clear eyed and matter of fact as the procession wheels by. "She's always been depressed," I hear her say to one of the police officers who have materialized to take statements—but the rest of her assessment is lost as I walk down the hall away from the trauma bay, back to the examination rooms where my first patient with the empty prescription is still waiting for me to come back.

As I approach, I can see this first patient's mom poking her head out the door impatiently, looking up and down the hall while talking on her cell phone, complaining loudly about the slow service and the amount of time she's been kept waiting in this horrible hospital. I expect to feel annoyed by these theatrics, but surprisingly, walking away from the chaos of the trauma bay, all I feel is a creeping sense of relief. Dubious and nonemergent as this task may be, here at least, is a patient I might actually be able to help.

* * *

After each stint I spend in the Peds ER I become more and more convinced of two things.

One: *The job of being a parent is just alternating between thankless cleanup and soul-crushing worry.* Of course, all we see in the Peds ER is the worst of it: the children who come to us are all sticky, oozing, squalling, and miserable; or else tremendously fragile—three-year-olds with cancer, toddlers with skull fractures, infants lethargic and depleted after just a day of dehydration, teenagers who impulsively chase a bottle of Tylenol with a fifth of vodka in an unfortunately effective effort to get their boyfriend's attention. How is it possible to be a parent and deal with the scope of all the things that could possibly go wrong? Not only the routine illnesses, but the vulnerability knowing that at any time, any of a thousand different disasters can befall even an otherwise healthy, well-cared-for child? How can they subject themselves to all that worry, the daily potential for heartbreak?

Two: *Parents are idiots.* I say this fully aware of how heartless it sounds, but honestly, after a long night in the Peds ER, rendered curmudgeonly by too much work and too little thanks, too much fatigue and not enough caffeine, I can't help myself. *Parents are idiots.* How can they let these things happen to their kids? How can they have such poor judgment? How can they be so utterly unable to distinguish what is normal from what is not? How can one parent *not* bring a child in for five days after a dog bite to the face, yet another parent bring their child by ambulance, urgent and demanding immediate medical attention, for a case of head lice? I know that not everyone went to medical school, and I don't expect them to come in naming their own diagnoses, but honestly, can't people exercise some *common sense?*

Teeming with the hubris endemic in those who don't actually have kids of their own, this is what I think during every shift in the Peds ER: *But with my own kids, it's going to be easy. I won't make the same mistakes these parents make. I'm a doctor, for chrissake, trained in pediatrics, even. When I have my own kids, I'll know exactly what to do.*

Fate apparently has a wicked sense of humor, because three weeks after finishing my ER rotation as a second-year Pediatrics resident, I am surprised to find out that I am pregnant.

5 · TRANSITIONS

A Change in Our Regularly Scheduled Programming

IRONICALLY, AT ROUGHLY THE SAME TIME that I find out that I am going to have a child of my own, I am making the final moves toward leaving the field of pediatric medicine entirely.

I was about halfway through my first year of Pediatrics residency when I started to get a sneaking suspicion that I had made the wrong decision by going into pediatrics in the first place. It wasn't that I didn't like pediatric patients—I did, and in fact, the idea of taking care of adult patients filled me with a sort of primitive dread. (The body hair! The smells! The yellowed, curling toenails! The general lack of mitigating cuteness!) It wasn't that I didn't like my colleagues—far the opposite, in fact; pediatricians as a whole are some of the nicest doctors you'll ever meet, with a natural nurturing sensibility and a tendency toward squeals and spontaneous hugging. And it wasn't that I didn't like the medicine—pediatric pathophysiology was in my opinion far more interesting than what I saw during my rotations in adult medicine, particularly with the range of disease processes we got to see at Columbia, the top center of academic pediatrics in the city. It was just that in those long, dark winter months, after Christmas and before it seems like the sun will ever shine again, I started to get this uncomfortable, niggling sense that *this is not what I am supposed to be doing with my life.*

I admit that part of it was flu season. As sort of an annual tradition, like some sort of electronic harbinger of doom, the children's hospital would send out an e-mail to all staff around late October or early November, heralding the first diagnosed case of influenza in the hospital. Cut through all the administrative admonitions for staff to get their flu shots and the usual epidemiological details about viral strains, and this e-mail in effect amounted to an alarm to BATTEN DOWN THE HATCHES, FLU SEASON IS HERE. And so for the next five months, the Pediatrics staff was essentially under siege, the ER overflowing with vomiting, coughing, crying children; clinic waiting rooms filled to capacity with walk-in patients; with most of the residents, our puny immune systems rendered insensible with fatigue, no match for the virulent and often projectile nature of these bugs. War is hell, but flu season in a Pediatrics hospital should at least count as one of the outer circles of Dante's inferno.

I can deal with flu season in and of itself—after all, getting sick while working with children is to be expected, and I don't mind sick children or their parents as a rule. It's just the tedium of the day-to-day, seeing the same few things over and over and over again, repeating the catechism *fluids, bland diet, Tylenol* until the process of seeing patients starts to feel more like working on an assembly line than practicing medicine. I don't like this automated feeling, and never want to feel like my patients are just a pile of charts to work through, a looming stack of work to be done. I just don't *enjoy* myself. And plus, there's always that fear lurking in the background that the numbing effect of repetition is dulling my nascent medical instincts. Certainly, ninety-nine out of a hundred vomiting children in the dead of January will have some manner of virus, and be effectively treated with the *fluids, bland diet, Tylenol* litany. But one of them may have something different, something more serious, something camouflaged under the brush-and-rifle fire of the ninety-nine other essentially healthy children. *Did I miss that one diagnosis?* I think every night. *Was I too quick to write off that kid as gastroenteritis when he may in fact have some sort of metabolic disorder or intestinal obstruction? Was I in too much of a rush, just because I had three more patients waiting in my chart box and probably fifteen more crowding around the reception desk waiting for walk-in appointments?* The question niggles at me every day; I'm feeling guilty at not being able to devote as much time or attention to each patient as I would like to, yet the next day feeling the same pressure to *go go go, move move move* the patients through yet again, back on the assembly line and unable to do anything about it.

But maybe this is just a product of residency. Certainly, residents are the workhorses of the hospital, so understandably we are under pressure, feel rushed and often unfulfilled. And maybe it is just to be expected that as a first-year resident, so much of what I am doing from day to day is completely removed from medicine itself. After morning rounds on the wards, I spend hours on the phone with social workers, faxing forms to insurance companies and pharmacies, transcribing the verbal orders that attendings give into the computerized medical order system that the hospital uses, then running around afterward dogging the poor nurses, checking that these orders are carried out before afternoon rounds. "I need a secretary," I often joke with the other residents, as I fly around the wards with a ragged sheaf of papers, more forms and requisitions sticking out of the pockets of my increasingly stained and wrinkled lab coat. But the truth of it is, if I actually *had* a nonmedical assistant to help me with the purely clerical aspects of my day-to-day work, what would I have left to do? As it is, probably only 10 percent of my daily routine is spent directly at a patient's bedside, doing procedures or conducting physical exams. The other 90 percent of the time, I am doing mindless administrative work—on the computer, over the phone, at the fax machine. *This is why I went to medical school?* I ask myself. *This is why I became a doctor?*

But ultimately, what pushes me to decide to leave

pediatrics is that when I try to envision myself ten years from now, for all the agonizing and my desire to stay my present course, I cannot conceive of a career within pediatrics that will keep me vital and excited for the rest of my life. I know that I enjoy working with sick patients, relish the excitement of hospital-based acute care (as opposed to clinic-based primary care and health maintenance), and like to do procedures; but cycling through all my options for specialty training—pediatric cardiology, pediatric intensive care, pediatric emergency medicine—nothing seems like quite the right fit.

Additionally, the flexibility of my chosen field is of critical importance to me. I know that I want a career in medicine, but I also know that Joe and I are looking forward to having a family, and being able to provide the balance between home and work that such a commitment deserves. Looking at some of my Pediatrics attendings even in subspecialty fields—there at all hours, working weekends, running ragged even many years or sometimes decades into their careers—I fear that instead of a balanced life, I will end up having to choose one side or the other.

I realize now in retrospect that I made a classic medical-student mistake when I chose to go into Peds. I confused my hobby with my career. *I like children*, I had thought, *I like playing with children, like taking care of children, I think childhood disease processes are interesting, so why* shouldn't *I like Peds?* Now I understand better. I like children, I like being a doctor, but that doesn't make me a pediatrician.

So quietly, guiltily, I start exploring some of my other options. It is a decision that I have put off for a long time, because in my limited experience, switching fields once you were already in residency simply *wasn't done*, and in defecting from one field to another you were simultaneously branding yourself both a quitter *and* a traitor. But the fact of it is that people *do* switch fields, and if you start asking around, it's surprising just how many people have. Internists who decide to go into psychiatry. Emergency medicine doctors who switch into radiology. Surgeons who bag it all and go to business school. Some people finish entire residencies and then start completely new ones from scratch, guided by things like academic interest, market forces, or (like me) the realization of wrong decisions made coming out of medical school. But it *is* done. And those who switch are generally happy with their choices, most of them made after the naïveté of med school has worn off and a real understanding of what it is to have a career in medicine, and what our options truly are, has set in.

Tammy, a coresident who has come to the same conclusions as I have and has elected to switch into an Anesthesia residency in Boston, encourages me to look into anesthesiology as well, pointing out that the field offers many of the things I'm looking for in a medical career. Anesthesiology is completely hands-on, she tells me, it's front-line medicine, it's acute care, it's exciting, the practitioners are happy, and frankly, the job market after graduation is excellent and offers options for a variety of lifestyles, both for the workaholic and the practitioner juggling medicine and family. So after some research on my own, another round of applications, and some interdepartmental negotiations between the two programs, I am accepted as a resident in the Anesthesiology Department at Columbia-Presbyterian. I will finish out my second year of Pediatrics residency and will start training in anesthesia on July 1, 2005.

Which is why it came as a little of a surprise when a few months later, I found out that I was pregnant. My due date? July 26, 2005.

So maybe our timing was not ideal.

* * *

Some would argue that you probably shouldn't have a baby during residency at all. Few might come out and say so, but one thing we know for sure: the good folks at the dog pound surely would not approve.

Early in my third year of medical school, I had decided that I wanted to get a dog. Actually, I can pinpoint the exact date: September 12, 2001. It was really the culmination of thwarted dog desire that I'd been culturing my entire life—as a child, I'd begged my parents time and time again for a dog, only to be told that the only way this would ever happen is if I found a dog that could feed and walk itself. (Somehow, I never managed to find a breed that could satisfy these conditions.) After college, I figured that I was finally an adult and therefore free to get a dog of my own, but by then I was a med student with no free time and even less free space. Somehow the moment just didn't seem quite right.

However, in the days after 9/11, the idea of putting off *anything* enjoyable suddenly seemed like a ridiculous notion. After all, they flew planes into our buildings, we were at war, and for all I knew, the world could end tomorrow. The least I could do is to get a *dog,* for god's sake. Why wait? Would there even *be* a later? George Bush was standing on a pile of rubble with a bullhorn! If I didn't get a dog, then the terrorists would win! (This all seemed to make sense at the time.)

Coincidentally, there was a flyer hanging in the lobby of the medical school building advertising eight-week-old cocker spaniel puppies for sale. I called the number listed and made arrangements to go inspect the litter. The owner, Ray, a virologist in one of the university research labs, agreed to pick me up in front of the building later that afternoon and take me to his apartment down on Riverside Drive, where he said the puppies and their mother were temporarily taking residence.

"Hold on—you called a *strange man* and got in his *car* to go to his *apartment* because he said he had some *puppies* there?" Joe spluttered in disbelief upon my eventual return. "What are you, five years old? Did he promise you candy too? Haven't you heard of Stranger Danger?" So perhaps getting into his car wasn't the most careful move on my part, but in fact, he did take me to his apartment and indeed, there was a litter of straw-colored puppies there, soft and squirmy and absolutely adorable. I lay there on the linoleum, letting the puppies crawl all over me, mentally checking my meager checkbook balance and wondering if it would be possible to take them all. But then I realized that I was a medical student living in an apartment with three roommates with whom I hadn't even discussed the possibility of dog ownership (one of them, I think, was actually allergic to dogs), and cooler heads prevailed. So I didn't get a puppy that day. But I didn't give up the idea either.

A year later, during our final year of medical school, Joe and I were living together in an apartment downtown. (We were not scheduled to get married until the following spring, but my parents gave us the go-ahead to cohabitate just so long as we didn't tell my eighty-year-old grandmother.) Now, with no roommates and two responsible adults to split up the work, surely we could get a puppy. We drove to a dog pound on Long Island one weekend in November. And drove back empty-handed.

Turns out that the people at the animal shelter didn't think that medical students made very good dog owners. The screening process, which entailed an application and two phone references, who were called while we waited outside the door trying to look like we weren't listening, was fairly rigorous, and when they called us back to the adoption desk, we knew that we'd failed. Apparently, per dictum of the shelter, no one was allowed to adopt a puppy if they were planning to be out of the house for more than two hours at a time over the next ten months. This limited the population of acceptable puppy adopters to unemployed agoraphobics and bedbound invalids, and thus we were counseled to adopt an older, housebroken dog. This narrowed down our shelter picks from about a hundred animals to one, an eight-year-old pit bull named Kronis who, while house-trained, also looked as though he was considering a tasty meal of nails and broken glass, after which point he would kill me in my sleep. So we didn't get a puppy that day either.

We eventually went back to the same animal shelter about a month later and *did* end up adopting a nine-week-old puppy, a black Labrador mix that we named Cooper. How did we get around the restrictive covenant at the shelter? Well, I'm not proud to tell you, but—*we lied.* No two ways about it, I looked the adoption volunteer in the eye and told them that while it was true, my husband was a medical student (this much they already had on file from our previous failed application), I had since graduated and was now taking some time off to be a freelance writer who worked from home. Why, of *course* I had time to raise and train a puppy. Didn't I mention that I work from home? In fact, I rarely leave the house, except to venture out to one of the many fine parks and dog runs in our neighborhood. Which I can do, because I work from home. Our references were coached to say the same thing, and if the adoption counselors noted the wooden recitation of our seemingly perfect qualifications for puppy ownership, they didn't say a thing.

And so we became a family of three. And despite the fact that we had been somewhat fast and loose with the truth, the fact of it was that, as fourth-year medical students, we actually *did* have a lot of free time for a new puppy. Though we did work long hours occasionally, between the two of us, Cooper was lavished with attention in the ways that only pets of a childless couple can truly be, admired and doted on in that *"Oh look, she thinks she's people"* kind of way. She was a dog, but we treated her like a baby because she was our practice for the real thing.

So while the dog shelter had rejected our application to adopt a baby dog because we worked too hard, we are now working even longer hours than before and getting ready to bring a baby human into the mix—though this time with no counseling or screening process whatsoever. The irony of this situation is not lost on me.

* * *

People decide to have children when they feel the time is right. But just when would that be?

During medical school, Joe and I discussed just this issue. When *would* the best time be for us to start our family? Medical school did not seem ideal—aside from the fact that we were studying all the time, living in university housing, and basically penniless, we just weren't ready. Having a baby during residency seemed like it would be even worse, as there would be no other time when our jobs held us so mercilessly and time-consumingly hostage. How would we have time to spend with the baby, with each other? For that matter, how would we be able to *afford* having a baby then? Though we would officially be a two-income household, the pay during residency isn't known for its munificence, and in any case, we'd be working so many hours that the salary was almost beside the point. No, we decided, it was probably better to wait until after training. *Later.* We would have kids later.

From years and years of practice, those of us in medical training have been indoctrinated to the lifestyle of delayed gratification. We spend all of our twenties and a significant portion of our thirties working very hard with very little to show for it outside of experience, all for the promise that some vague day in the future, things are going to fall into line. We will finish training, *then* start living our lives. *Until you're finished with your medical training,* we're told in ways both subtle and not so subtle, *everything else can wait.* And this is how things are prioritized. Hospital first, self second.

A few months before I found out that I was pregnant, I was on the general wards of the Pediatric medical service, rushing to gather patient lab results for afternoon rounds. Sitting next to me was one of the senior residents, who looked uncharacteristically glum. "It's crazy, this life we lead," he said out of nowhere, talking to no one in particular. Since I was the one sitting closest to him, I felt obligated to respond in some way. "Yeah? What do you mean?"

He turned to me, looking troubled. "I just found out yesterday that my fiancée's dad died."

"Oh." Though I turned away from the computer screen to look at him, I kept my hands on the keyboard, lest anyone close me out of my program. "I'm really sorry, man, that sucks."

"No," he said, looking distant, "what *sucks* is that when she told me, the first thing I thought, I mean the *first thing*, was, 'How in the world am I supposed to get a day off from the wards to go to this funeral?' Not about her dad, not about her, but about *work*." He looked down, puffed out his cheeks, and exhaled loudly. "I mean, how fucked up is *that*? How is it that work is the first thing we always think about?" Though I wanted to make him feel better, I couldn't disagree with him. Residency, after a period of months and years, takes your priorities, your perspective, your sense of normal and not normal, and tweaks it, such that you start to look at everything as though through a prism and start wondering why everyone else seems to be walking sideways.

It is easy to let medicine become a cult: to let it ruin your life, dictate all of your decisions and separate you from the other important things in your life. It is easy to lay blame on a job that is so all consuming. What better excuse really, than a profession cloaked in the virtues of altruism? Some of the best doctors I've ever worked with have indeed eschewed the luxuries of an outside life for the greater good of medicine, almost monastic in their devotion to their work and their patients. They live in the hospital, sometimes literally, with sleeping couches and several changes of clothes in their offices. They work nights, holidays, weekends, stay late, arrive early. By choice, medicine is their life. Everything else would only be a distraction. But it is unrealistic to think that we can all live up to that standard, nor do I necessarily think that we should aspire to it.

And really, when it comes to having children, what *would* be the "right" time? *Is* there a right time? Residency is brutal to be sure, but being a young attending isn't much better. And so people wait until later, until they're established, until they've built up a practice, until they've paid back their medical school debt; it is not infrequent to hear that people have waited so long for "the perfect time" that their window to have children has closed entirely.

Life is bigger than what the trajectory of our medical careers will allow. And just because medicine tries to consume our entire lives doesn't mean we have to willingly hand them over. And so the fall of 2004, after a rejuvenating and unfortunately too-short trip to Hawaii, Joe and I find out that I am pregnant.

It is a surprise, and even if we had planned this as an act of self-sabotage, the timing could not have been worse. All the same, we could not be happier.

* * *

One night, a few months before my due date, I am transporting a critically ill child from the ER to the Pediatric ICU when I bump into John, one of the third-year Pediatrics residents. He and his wife are new parents as well, having just had their first son about four months ago.

"Hey, John," I say cheerily, glad to be out of the ER and eager to prolong any interaction that might delay my return there. "How's it going up here tonight?"

"Meh," John replies apathetically.

"How's the baby?" I ask.

John turns to me, his hair rumpled, the lines of his face smudged with fatigue. "I haven't slept more than two hours at a stretch for the past four-and-a-half months."

"What? *Still?*" In my own naïve, still-childfree mind, I have this notion (though *fantasy* may be more accurate a word) that babies magically start sleeping through the night at around four months. Not to mention the fact that they are unceasingly adorable and smiley and can often be found flopping into piles of soft, fluffy towels like Snuggle, the fabric softener bear.

"Sleep now while you can," John intones sonorously, like the ghost of Jacob Marley, forgetting entirely that as a resident, the amount of sleep I can get is utterly out of my control, not to mention the fact that sleep, unlike canned goods, is not a commodity that can be stockpiled for later. "Also, don't breastfeed if you ever want to sleep again."

"I won't tell the general Peds establishment that you just said that out loud, John." I pause, thinking. "Anyway, it's not like *you* have to get up. *You* don't have the boobs."

"Yeah, but I hear him. I wake up anyway."

"But it's not the same for you as for your wife."

John has to concede on this point. "True. I don't know how women do it. Women are strong."

"Is your wife working too?" This cuts to the heart

of my concern. Being a resident is hard enough. Having a baby is hard enough. How am I supposed to do both at the same time?

"Naw, she's a lawyer," replies John, making a vague wave of his hand, which I suppose was intended to illustrate the field of law in all its complexities. "She's taking six months off to be with the baby. Though now I think she's going to extend it to nine months."

"Nine *months*! Wow, it's nice that she can do that before going back to work."

"Yeah." John is starting to fade again, eyelids heavy. "How long are you taking off when you squeeze out your piglet?"

"Oh, probably the standard resident maternity leave. Six weeks. I mean, you know. If they'll let me."

"Right. The standard."

And at this moment, I am suddenly filled with an unspeakable premonitory dread. Am I *really* going to do this? Am I really going to have a baby and start a new residency—a career move not known for its restorative effects on the sleep-deprived psyche—*at the same time?* Am I *nuts?* What the hell am I *thinking?* "Wow," I manage to say, once I unglue my tongue from the roof of my mouth, which has suddenly become alarmingly dry. "This next year is going to be really hard, isn't it?"

John, not much one for false assurances, looks at me stone-faced, and says, "Yes." The resounding postscript, *Dumbass*, is not spoken aloud—it doesn't need to be.

* * *

The last time I took care of a kid was about a year ago. Joe and I were babysitting for his sister's two-year-old son while she ran some errands, and the task seemed easy enough—especially since the kid was actually asleep when she left the house. Babysitting a toddler? Piece of cake. I settled on the couch and opened a book.

The problem was, the kid had the temerity to wake up, and it was all downhill from there. Joe's sister came home not two hours later to find her son rumpled, his diaper askew and covered in a fine dusting of neon orange crumbs from the Goldfish crackers I fed him for dinner. I was frazzled and covered in dog hair. Joe backed away cautiously as though the kid were radioactive, and feigned a sudden interest in the view out the window.

"Gee, I would think that two *doctors* would be able to take care of a two-year-old boy," drawled Joe's sister sarcastically after the shock wore off.

"Well," I countered, "I never said we were *good* doctors."

Of course, I have *taken care* of children before—after all, as a Pediatrics resident, I am around children every day. But what I come to realize is that despite my guise of expertise, what I actually do as a Pediatrics resident involves more writing orders and giving instructions for *others* to actually take care of my patients than it involves real-life childcare skill.

Apparently I am not the only one with this gap in experience. One of my attendings once told me that, after three years of Pediatrics residency and two years of private practice, she and her husband finally had a child of their own, only to realize upon their first day home from the hospital that she had no idea how she was supposed to bathe the baby. Should she just...pour water on him? Dunk him into the water like a teabag? What kind of soap should she use? Towel or blow-dryer? (*"I* don't know!" she recalls wailing to her husband, who was dumbfounded that his pediatrician wife couldn't seem to figure out how to get her own child clean. "The *nurse* usually does *that* part! Baby bathing was not covered on my Board exam!")

I have my own questions about dealing with a child of my own. For instance, one of the most basic issues of all is what I am supposed to do when the baby cries. Oh, a crying baby, the world's most piteous sound, one that I am more accustomed to provoking than placating. My current strategy for dealing with crying babies at work is as follows:

PLAN A:

Coo, "Oh, you want to go back to Mommy!" (or Daddy, as the case may be) and then pass off the screaming pink thing as fast as humanly possible to the waiting arms of the responsible adult. Hopefully the *real* experts know what to do. However, if no parents are around...

PLAN B:

Swaddle the kid up. Swaddling is something I actually have some degree of expertise in, having swaddled dozens, no, *hundreds*, of infants in the newborn nursery after their initial intake and exit exams. Sometimes this swaddling business makes the noises stop. Sometimes. If I have the time and resources, I occasionally also...

PLAN C:

Stick a pacifier in the kid's mouth. With the idea that they're supposed to...pacify...aren't they? However, when all else fails, as it frequently does...

PLAN D:

Walk over to the kid's nurse and say, "I don't know what I did, but he's all upset in there. Maybe he's hungry or something." Then walk away under the guise of having urgent doctorly business to take care of instead of copping to total incompetence.

Obviously, none of these strategies is going to work with my own kid. And there are other elementary things that I don't actually know how to do. For instance, how does one actually feed a baby? Burp a baby? Cut a baby's nails? The nurses usually do all that, and seem to have such a good handle on these things that I never really stopped and paid attention to what they were doing or how they were doing it. And good lord, the *crying*, what if I can't figure out what to do and our baby doesn't stop crying? *Ever?* Will his little head just explode?

As a doctor, I feel I should know these things. I *should*, but I don't. I suppose, like with everything else, I'll just pick it up on the job.

July Redux

As it turns out, I start both of my new jobs in the month of July, when I cross over, both figuratively and physically, the glowing glass skybridge connecting Children's Hospital to Milstein Hospital, where I begin my training in Anesthesia. The adult hospital, which has 745 beds, not only dwarfs my former stomping grounds but also thankfully sports far fewer creepy 1970s-era animal-motif murals. On the academic calendar, it's a time of transitions—once again, it's July, and I'm on unfamiliar turf in a completely new realm, bumbling and useless again, trying to figure out what the hell I'm supposed to be doing.

Almost no one outside of medicine (and even many people within it) knows what it is that anesthesiologists actually *do*. Sure, people understand that it has something to do with "putting people to sleep" during surgery, and most women understand that anesthesiologists and epidurals go hand in hand on the Labor and Delivery floor. But other than that, people generally have no idea of what it is that an anesthesiologist is really doing back there, secreted behind the surgical drapes, or what kind of training the specialty entails. Or, as my father-in-law once asked, "So, when you're giving anesthesia, is there a *doctor* in the room too?"

Anesthesiology is the field of medicine that concerns itself with the total care of the patient undergoing surgery. We put the patients to sleep, intubate them if necessary, provide pain relief and amnesia through a variety of pharmacologic agents, and basically run the equivalent of an intensive care unit consisting of one patient during the surgical procedure, providing support for breathing and blood pressure, administering medications and blood transfusions as needed. And when the shit hits the fan in the operating room, it often falls to the anesthesiologist to make sure that the patient survives.

For me, though, coming from pediatrics, one of the true beauties of anesthesiology is that when you're in that operating room and your patient is on the table, that's it. That's your one patient, the only patient in the world so far as you're concerned, where all your efforts and attention can be focused. There aren't twenty-five other patients on the floor waiting to be rounded on. There aren't patients stacked in the waiting room knocking down your door. There aren't nurses paging you about Mr. Jones, the patient you've never met before but are cross-covering for another resident, who wants to talk to a doctor now about the results of his lung biopsy, and who incidentally wants to know if he can walk down to the first floor for a smoke. It's just you and your patient, and you are attuned to his every need, every beat of his heart, every breath he takes. And if your patient needs something? Medication for his blood pressure? Treatment for his arrhythmia? A central line through which to infuse a vasoactive drip? Well, that's you too. No writing the order for the nurse to carry out three hours later. No calling for another medical consultant to come steal all the fun. No writing a prescription and seeing the patient three months later to learn that he was never even able to get it filled because he lost his insurance coverage. It's real-time medicine, and you're the one providing it, right here, right now.

People are fooled into thinking that anesthesiologists have it easy, because when things are going well, it doesn't look like we are doing much of anything. Standing next to a patient, watching a monitor, fiddling with dials, occasionally pushing medication through the IV. What's so hard about that? With experience, the best anesthesia practitioners can make it look effortless, but all it takes to shatter the illusion is to watch a first-year Anesthesiology resident in July trying to manage a patient.

As a Pediatrics resident, I found that in general, it is relatively difficult to kill a patient, or even to hurt them too badly. Barring unusual and thankfully rare circumstances, a seriously ill pediatric patient gives you some time to realize that they are sick, and unless you have missed a series of important diagnostic signs that herald some grievous injury or infection, or are willfully malevolent (pushing large doses of a toxic medication or smothering some kid with a pillow in the night perhaps), imperiling children while practicing general pediatrics is difficult to do. In contrast, to hurt someone while administering anesthesia is actually fairly easy. There are just *so many ways* that things can go wrong. Even things so simple as forgetting to flip a switch, turning a dial down when you meant to turn it up, misreading a medication label. It is nerve-wracking to say the least—*I can't believe they're letting me do this,* I think on many occasions—and for months into my Anesthesia residency, I worry that each case I perform will end up with Grandma leaving the room in a box.

The July of my first year of Anesthesia residency, I feel like a medical student again, and not even a very smart one. In Pediatrics at least, I made my bones. I was a good resident, rotated as a senior on the wards, spent five months in the ICU, and established myself as a good doctor with solid instincts and a strong work ethic. Now, I feel like everything I have learned in the last two years had been worthless. *The childhood immunization schedule?* Useless. *Issues in enteral feeding of the premature infant?* Useless. *The appropriate developmental age at which a child can talk, walk, use a pincer grasp or build a tower of five blocks?* Blank stares all around. Not only is all the expertise I gained in the past two years obsolete, I have actually forgotten all the useful elements of *adult* medicine that I learned in medical school. I spend the first few months of my Anesthesia residency wandering through the hospital in a low-grade panic. *My next patient is a ninety-eight-year-old woman? Is this a typo? I didn't know people even* lived *to be ninety-eight years old. It says here in the chart that she has Alzheimer's? What am I supposed to do about that?*

But there will be plenty of time for those details later. My first month, in July, I merely apply myself to understanding the basics of the practice of anesthesia. Which medications I should give when. How the anesthesia machine works. How exactly I am supposed to intubate someone, and what the vocal cords look like. Everything I am doing is completely new to me. I have absolutely no idea where anything is, what I am doing, anything about the basic etiquette of the operating room. I am a disaster.

My one saving grace is that the Anesthesia Department, perhaps out of pity, allows me to spend the first month of my residency doing pediatric anesthesia, so at least the patient population is familiar—some of them I have actually taken care of only a few weeks ago on the wards. The other small mercy is that the attending who has been assigned to supervise me one-on-one, Dr. Ingrid Fitz-James, is also a pediatrician-turned-anesthesiologist. And though she is intense to work with and has a, shall we say, *decisive* way of communicating what exactly it is that you are doing wrong, she is an excellent and patient teacher once you prove to her that you are serious, that you are reasonably intelligent, and that, for all your mistakes, you are *trying*. I spend those first few weeks basically dogging her every move, soaking in so much information so quickly that at the end of each day, I can literally feel my brain throbbing. Or maybe that's just from the anesthetic gas I am inadvertently taking in all day.

Not being familiar with the new work environment, I try not to call attention to the fact that I am nine months pregnant, but even in baggy scrubs, that fact is a little difficult to hide. As a first-year resident, I want to keep a low profile, working extra hard and not asking for any special favors and, probably overcompensating for the fact that I know I will be taking a few weeks off less than a month into my new residency. But Dr. Fitz-James (whose husband is a high-risk obstetrician) will have none of it, kicking me out of the OR for bathroom breaks and stopping just short of force-feeding me between cases. When she notices my ankles, swollen after a long day on my feet, she procures a pair of compression stockings from the supply room, which she then shoos me into the locker room with to put on under my scrub pants. "You have to take care of yourself," she admonishes me, playing mother hen under the guise of mentorship. "You'll never be a good anesthesiologist if you don't take care of your body."

Toward the end of my first month, we are starting our last case of the day, a thirteen-year-old boy having a laparoscopic appendectomy. We are in the operating room with him when Dr. Fitz-James makes an unexpected announcement. "Dr. Au," (she calls all the residents "Doctor," occasionally sarcastically, though not in this particular instance) "you are going to be doing this case on your own." She says this, of course, after the patient is asleep and his mother has left the room. I hold the mask over my patient's face, my fingertips gripping under the bony shelf of his mandible, Dr. Fitz-James making some slight adjustments to my hand position and watching me as I squeeze the bag, filling the boy's lungs with anesthetic gas. She watches me flip open the laryngoscope with a satisfying metallic *click*, pantomiming in front of me how she wants me to stand, hold my arm, keeping my back straight and my legs slightly crouched. She stands by as I slip the blade in, sweeping the patient's tongue as she has showed me, and when I tell her that I can see the vocal cords, she hands me what I need so I do not have to lose my view fumbling for the endotracheal tube, and says emphatically (she is almost always emphatic), *"Go for it."* And I do.

The tube slides in easily. The clear plastic fogs with condensation as the patient's chest rises under the gentle pressure from my reservoir bag. Carbon dioxide exits his lungs and is confirmed on my monitors. "You're on your own, kiddo," she says with a nod after the tube's position is confirmed, and sure enough, true to her word, she moves away, making herself inconspicuous in the corner of the room. She is still physically there, and I know that she will be quick to respond in case of any emergency, but I understand that I am to act as though I am alone. She is trying to teach me to work independently. She is trying to teach me to be an anesthesiologist.

I look at the patient, look at my monitors. The surgery is about to commence. I adjust a few things, give a little push of pain medication. The incision is smooth, and the patient stays stable. We are under way.

The administration of general anesthesia is often compared to flying a plane. There are the crucial points analogous to takeoff and landing, namely the induction of anesthesia with intubation, along with the emergence from anesthesia and extubation. There is also the maintenance phase of anesthesia, which I have taken to calling the "in-flight movie." With a stable patient and a smooth surgical course, the maintenance phase occurs without much event. Constant vigilance is always called for, of course, but with some experience, anesthesiologists can relax during the maintenance phase, all while keeping one ear and one eye out for trouble. As a novice, however, I am incapable of relaxing, and constantly dart my eyes back and forth between the surgical field, my monitors, my machine, the patient. *Is everything going OK? Is the patient feeling any pain? Should I give him some more pain medication or turn up the gas? There's some bleeding on the field, but is that too much bleeding? How's his blood pressure? His oxygenation?*

At some point, my heart still racing with rookie adrenaline, I turn my head to Dr. Fitz-James (who is pretending to read a book in the corner), grin excitedly at her from under my mask, and say excitedly, "I'm flying the plane!" Without looking up, she raises her eyebrows in an *I can't hear you because I'm not here* expression, but I can tell that she is pleased.

And that's how it all starts. You start requiring so much support, a teacher literally bodily guiding you through the motions, *your hand here, your head here, look at this, feel that,* and day by day, month by month, you feel more comfortable, start to do more on your own, pick up tricks and lessons from different people to cobble together into your own practice. It doesn't happen overnight and we start practically from scratch, but the amazing thing is that almost all of us get there. It is medicine's way of replenishing its own pool. The old guard training and grooming the new. Young doctors transitioning into new roles and learning as they go.

In an academic hospital, that's just how it goes in July.

* * *

A few weeks later, I am still learning about anesthesia, though this time from the other end. I am back in Children's Hospital, though now on the Labor and Delivery floor, hunched over on my hospital bed in position to receive my labor epidural.

As a former Pediatrics resident and a current Anesthesia resident, I am in the rare position of having been intimately familiar with the Labor and Delivery floor well before I had cause to be there as a patient myself. Many nights while working in the Neonatal ICU, I would be called to assist in a delivery, usually to examine or resuscitate sick newborns in distress. I hope I will not require the consultation of any of my former Pediatrics classmates in that respect, but welcome the services of my Anesthesia colleagues, as an anesthesia-free birth is not one that I ever really considered. (I am of the school of thought, radical though it may be, that pain is a bad thing.) And so here I am, hunched over a pillow with the back of my gown untied, getting my lower back scrubbed off with cold antiseptic Betadine.

"Should I expect to feel any problems breathing with the epidural in?" I ask the Anesthesia attending, who is standing behind me fussing with the pieces of the epidural kit. I am just trying to make conversation, and this is something I think I recall from the chapter on regional anesthesia I just finished reviewing.

There is a pause. "You don't know much about epidural anesthesia, do you?" the attending barks, which I think is sort of a nonanswer. Normally, I would be flustered and abashed, sneaking off later to flip through my textbook and review the chapter on epidural anesthesia, but today I don't really care. I'm not here as a resident, I'm here as a patient. I can figure out the right answer later.

Though every source on the matter told me different, I find my labor to actually be fairly enjoyable. I know everything is relative, but all I could think of was, *I'm lying in bed! During the* day! *During the* work *day! And I am watching TV! And even though I'm at the hospital, no one needs me to do* anything! Labor is awesome. Labor is like being on vacation. I wish I could be in labor forever. Joe, dressed in scrubs, having come in straight from clinic, joins me, and together we watch *The Tony Danza Show.* Since when does Tony Danza have a daytime talk show? He really *is* the boss.

Fortunately no one takes my desire to be in labor forever too seriously, not even my own body. But what I realize when the time comes is this: everyone talks about "pushing" the baby out, and anyone knows it involves a lot of effort and maybe sweating and cursing, but how exactly do you push? I have no idea. Push how? Push *who*? It is not as obvious as I once figured.

As a Pediatrics resident I got called to so many deliveries where I felt like I was standing there at the foot of the bed for *days* because the mom was giving what looked to be the wimpiest little pushes, to the point that everyone in attendance—including the baby—eventually started to get kind of irritable. Finally, what would invariably happen was that the obstetrician would just whip out the vacuum or forceps and *drag* that kid out of there, because after two hours smashed in the birth canal, most babies decided they didn't like this "being born" business very much *at all*, which would manifest as some unhappy-looking dips on the fetal heart rate monitor. And meanwhile, through all this, as the Pediatrics resident waiting for *my* patient to emerge for the handoff, I'd just be standing there with my little blue towel, tapping my feet, all the while thinking about the sandwich I could be eating *right now* if only the mom could just push with a little more *oomph*. But what I know now is that...pushing? Pushing is *hard*.

Cal is born with his eyes wide open. "He's big!" is the first thing my OB says, and I wholeheartedly agree. "He's so pink!" adds Joe, whose eyes are peeled for any signs of neonatal distress. But of course there are no such signs. Cal is wiggling and crying and I cannot help but instinctively calculate his one-minute Apgar score as a nine. The nurse towels off Cal briefly before placing him in my arms, and he looks up at me, a few minutes old and already *looking* at me, by god, the kid is a *genius*! He is vigorous and perfect and beautiful. And I think the same thing that

I thought the first time Dr. Fitz-James told me that I was going to do that case on my own. *This is unbelievable. I can't believe I'm allowed to do this. I can't believe I have the responsibility of taking care of this whole other person. I hope to god I know what I'm doing and don't screw this up.*

Cal has been dried and is squalling with the indignity of being placed on the scale. He has been wrapped up like a little burrito, the same way that I have wrapped scores and scores of other people's babies after examining them, and then he is handed off to Joe. Gently, as though Cal is made of blown glass, Joe takes the baby in his arms and kisses him lightly on the forehead. Cal, quiet and alert now, gazes straight up into his eyes. Joe looks over at me and, with one word, sums up everything I'm thinking.

"Wow."

* * *

"Honey, I'm a doctor, I should be able to install a car seat."

"Fine. Here, I'm going to take our baby out of the car seat first so you can mess with it without accidentally punching him in the face."

"OK, so I take this strap here, and I pull here, across here..."

"What happened?"

"Wait, let me start over."

"Hold on, you have the car seat backwards. It has to be facing the back of the car. Under twenty pounds or less than a year, they have to face the back of the car. Or something. That's just what I say to people when they leave the hospital, I've never actually applied this knowledge in real life."

"Fine, maybe it'll work better if it's facing the back. OK, pull strap here, through here, under this plastic wedge... *shit*."

"Don't curse in front of the baby! He might grow up emotionally scarred and end up getting a swastika tattooed on his neck."

"He doesn't even speak English yet."

"Do you need help? Maybe one of those security guard people know. Or wait, grab one of those Hasidic dads in the lobby, they have a million kids, they probably know how to do this."

"Honey, these are the hands of a *surgeon*. Trust me. I can put in a car seat. I just need more slack on this seat belt."

"OK."

"And maybe a nail gun."

"Is it too late to just take the subway home?"

* * *

Turns out that, compared to being a resident, taking care of a newborn is easy.

True, those first few weeks of parenting do bear some resemblances to residency—never quite feeling like you've gotten enough sleep, a general deterioration in personal hygiene and grooming, the tendency to be awakened in the middle of the night by high-pitched noises. However, unlike my pager, even when Cal wakes me up at three o'clock in the morning, he rarely does it to tell me about a new patient being admitted from the ER, or to ask me to change Mr. Grablowsky's dietary orders from Regular to Kosher. Also, I'm not biologically conditioned to love my pager. Having a newborn is like being on call every single day and night, but with no nurses or any other intermediaries, and only one patient on your roster, who you happen to adore beyond anything you could have possibly imagined. Maybe this is what concierge medicine is like.

As a mercy to his clueless parents, Cal is also relatively easy to take care of, as newborn babies go. Thankfully, many aspects of parenting are fairly intuitive. Cuddling and soothing your own baby is not something that many people need to be taught how to do. Feeding your baby—well, that must be encoded in the genome as well. Other things, however, take a little more on-the-job experience. For example, our first day home with Cal, about seven hours go by before I remember that babies wear diapers, and diapers occasionally need to be changed. I don't know what ultra-absorbent polymers they're packing into Pampers these days, but by the time I realize that I actually have to exchange wet diapers for dry ones, the diaper Cal is wearing has reached maximum capacity, swollen to the point of being virtually spherical. Luckily, Cal, ever-forgiving, doesn't seem to mind much.

Cal has a mild case of neonatal jaundice, for which, I know from my Pediatrics background, he has three risk factors: he has a different blood type from mine, he is breastfed, and he is Asian. (Well, half-Asian. Fine, two-and-a-half risk factors.) Neonatal jaundice, a yellowing of the skin and eyes caused by high levels of bilirubin in the bloodstream, is common, transient, and usually benign, but does require periodic blood draws in the first few days of life, until the baby's bilirubin levels start falling. Bilirubin levels exceeding a certain threshold can require admission to the hospital for phototherapy, which is, in essence, a stint on a baby tanning bed, as ultraviolet rays can help with bilirubin excretion in the urine. This is something that, over the course of my Pediatrics residency, I must have seen hundreds of times. As for the blood draws entailed, make that *thousands* of times. I had ordered blood draws on babies every single day for the last two years. I had performed the blood draws myself. I had enlisted the help of nurses, medical students, even the parents if they had the stomach for it, to hold down one squirming limb or other while I attempted to direct the gleaming, 22-gauge needle toward the purplish shadow that I hoped was the vein. This is all routine, right?

The first time I watch Cal get his blood drawn at the pediatrician's office, from a small vein in the back of his hand, I cry. I actually *cry* in the pediatrician's office, and I am so embarrassed that it only makes me cry more. In fact, Cal stops crying before I do. "Wow, maybe there is something to this hormone thing," Joe observes.

Over the course of the next few weeks of my maternity leave, I often think what a waste it is, all this insight into parenthood, *actual parenthood*, only *after* completing my training in pediatrics. What a better doctor I would be to those parents, now realizing the difference between focusing on one child, *your* child—for all intents and purposes the *only* child in the world you really care about—versus being torn between the care of many, many children, all of whom you are responsible for but none that actually belong to you. *I understand them now,* I think to myself as I catch myself fussily attending to Cal's rapidly desiccating umbilical stump, or scrutinizing the minute rise and fall of his chest, making sure that one breath follows the next. *I finally get it.* All those frantic calls at inconvenient hours, those late-night ER visits for nothing, all the mountains made out of molehills. *When it's your own kid, nothing is "just a virus" or "just a scratch." There is no more "just." When it's your own child,* everything *is important.*

My mother gave birth to me, her first child, in residency, which, as uncommon as it is now, was even *more* unthinkable then, in the 1970s. She took three weeks off for her maternity leave. My six-week maternity leave seems positively decadent in comparison, but flies by nonetheless in a dreamy haze of sweet downy-head smelling and itty-bitty toenail counting. But when my leave ends, I am confronted with the reality of the situation. I now have *two* full-time jobs—residency and parenthood—each of which demand my complete attention, almost all of my waking hours, and both of which society has drilled into me are my first, most important priorities. The stakes are huge. Half-assed efforts at either would be unacceptable.

Before Cal was born, I thought I was a pretty good doctor. Before I went back to work, I thought I was a pretty good parent. But when I had to do both at the same time, that illusion of competence all pretty much fell apart.

6. ANESTHESIA

IF THERE'S ONE THING that the long process of medical training has in spades, it's historical precedent. While plenty has changed in medicine over the past hundred years, there are also many things that have remained constant, and the process of training new medical school graduates is one of them. This is the process known as residency.

The residency system arose late in the nineteenth century. Originated by Dr. William Osler, the first physician-in-chief at the Johns Hopkins Hospital in Baltimore, the residency process was developed as a sort of prolonged apprenticeship for medical school graduates, in which newly minted doctors would work alongside their older, more seasoned colleagues, and in doing so gain the knowledge and skills necessary to practice specialty medicine independently. There are currently nineteen recognized types of medical residencies in the United States, requiring anywhere from three to seven years of postgraduate training.

The reason that young doctors were called residents in Osler's day was because residents lived in the hospital. Not just figuratively, but literally. There were banks of dormitory-style rooms with beds and desks, and food and laundry services were provided, so really there was no reason to ever leave. It was an ascetic lifestyle, spare and focused, the monastic qualities of which were only emphasized by the fact that women were largely barred from medical school.

Historically, complete devotion to the training process was not only expected, but required. In fact, around the turn of the century, some programs even forbade marriage, as they thought it a dangerous distraction from the all-consuming residency experience. While it was draconian, the old-school model effectively took care of the question of how resident physicians were to balance work with their outside lives: they weren't supposed to *have* outside lives.

But for all the drawbacks of medicine in that earlier age, there is something to envy. For residents in the early 1900s, their responsibilities were clear. They were there to learn medicine and take care of patients. Nothing else. When they had to stay late on the wards, there wasn't that niggling guilt, that heavy feeling in the chest, of knowing that someone outside the hospital who needed your care just as much was just going to have to wait. The residents back then had no outside responsibilities, they had no opposing interests to resolve. Those residents weren't supposed to be anywhere else but right there.

That must have been nice.

Reentry

The typical mother returning to a job outside of the home has to, at some point, accept the fact that she will be spending some time away from her baby. I have to come to terms with the fact that I will be spending a *lot* of time away from mine.

"I love you, you know," I tell Cal, that last week before returning to work. "Even when I'm not right here with you, I'm going to be thinking about you and waiting to come home so that I can be with you." Ever the pragmatist, Cal crosses his eyes, farts, then falls asleep.

My first task before returning to work (I try not to think of it as abandoning my newborn infant to the careless vagaries of an indifferent, cruel world, though at times, it feels *exactly* like this) is finding childcare. Our options on this front are somewhat limited. My parents both work full-time at their busy medical practices, and Joe's entire family is firmly entrenched in Ohio, so barring emergencies requiring a summoning of the grandparental cavalcade, we need to look outside our own families for the day-to-day care of our baby. Daycare is another option we cross off the list fairly quickly. Despite being one of the more affordable options and popular with many hospital employees, no daycare centers in the area are open anywhere near early enough—we estimate a

6:00 a.m. drop-off time—to accommodate the child of two parents who keep operating room schedules. (Well, there *is* that one "24-hour care facility," but upon reading their literature a little more in depth, I quickly realize that this is more of a "crisis nursery," to allow parents stressed to the limits of their capacity, psychic and otherwise, to drop off their children, sometimes for days, to decrease the temptation to throw said children out the window.)

So, no Grandma's house, no daycare—what we are left with is the realization that we will need to find a nanny to stay with Cal while we are at work. But how do you find a stranger to take care of your child? Someone whom you can *trust*? And, somewhat more pragmatically for us, how do you find someone who is willing to show up for work at 5:45 a.m. every morning, work twelve-hour days most days of the week, be flexible if (rather, *when*) we have emergencies at work that keep us away for hours at a time? Furthermore, how do you find someone who understands that, despite the fact that Joe and I are technically both doctors, we actually don't have very much money? And that while we are willing to pay up to 50 percent of our combined take-home pay for childcare, that still amounts to not very much? In short, we need to find someone who is willing to work resident hours for resident pay. And what kind of sane person would be willing to do *that*?

Eventually, we do manage to find someone who will fit the bill, a nanny we "inherit" from two other doctors at the hospital who are just completing their training and moving to the comparatively greener pastures of New Jersey. It will be a stretch for us financially, but she enables me to go back to work, at least, and seems willing to do her part. That is to say, she will keep Cal alive until either Joe or I return from work. Leaving for work that first day, I hustle out the door with a bright smile and an overloud cheerful voice, to disguise the fact that I am actually close to tears. I have essentially left the most important thing in my life in the care of a virtual stranger. *She* is going to take care of my baby and *I* am going to take care of other people. It is all cloaked in the illusion of altruism—I have to go back to being a doctor so that I can Help People—but then why is it that going back to work seems like the most selfish decision in the world? How does this make sense? What the hell am I doing?

My first day back from maternity leave, I am on twenty-four-hour overnight call. Back in the saddle again.

* * *

A few months into working motherhood, I discover something that surprises me. I am turning into a hippie mom.

I have always scorned hippie-mom types. It is not quite politically correct to say so, but I think crunchy granola moms are largely insane. Breastfeeding militants, anti-circumcisers, "natural birth" proponents (the term implying that those who opt for or end up needing medical interventions are somehow "unnatural") used to send me shuddering in the other direction. As a resident, walking into Labor and Delivery suites where mothers were writhing on a tie-dyed birthing ball while a doula was rubbing peppermint oil on their chests exasperated me, and it was hard not to roll my eyes. And don't get me started on those who refuse to immunize. The idea of parents turning their back on one of the greatest advances in modern medicine in some misguided effort to "save" their children from evil humors truly makes me see red. So no, I am no hippie-mom sympathizer. And yet, I have somehow become one.

It started with the circumcision issue. Before Cal was born, I didn't really care whether or not he got circumcised—what the hell, it's just some skin, who cares what happens to it—and deferred to Joe, the one parent who actually *had* a penis, to make the decision. Joe did not feel strongly either, but together we decided, whatever, we'd circumcise our son.

And then he was born. And he was *perfect*. And suddenly, it just seemed crazy to tempt fate. I mean, it's not like there's anything in medicine without risk. A circumcision is relatively low risk as procedures go, but without any strong religious or cultural imperative, why have the procedure at all? It serves no functional importance. There are no significant medical benefits. I'm not going to cause my baby pain for *that*. And so we didn't circumcise our son. It was the gateway drug.

Next came the breastfeeding. I knew from the outset that I was going to at least give breastfeeding the old college try, but I honestly didn't know how long I would be able to keep it up after I started back at work, because really, how many times a day would I be able to pump? I was a medical resident, it's not like I had time or an office or even a door that I could close. I rented a breast pump, but only for a three-month trial, figuring that I probably wouldn't continue to breastfeed much beyond that.

What I didn't realize was how much I would love it. I didn't think I would, but I do. I have always been one of those people who get vaguely squeamish when I see women breastfeeding in public—especially older toddlers—but I just *love* the feeling of that perfect little circle formed by me and my baby. The warm snuffles, the tiny soft hands on my shirt, the insular little world created between the two of us. This, after so many hours spent away from home, was what both Cal and I craved. So I pumped at work. Anytime I could find time, I pumped. And when I came home, I breastfed seemingly constantly.

Finally, there was the matter of sleeping. Early on, when Cal was born, we set him up in a small portable crib, which we kept next to our bed. Our expectation was that he'd sleep there for the immediate newborn period and then at some point move to the sturdy wood crib in his own room, where he would of course sleep through the night all on his own, like a baby in a diaper commercial.

There were two things I didn't realize. One is that, as both a resident and the mother of a very young infant, I was beyond exhausted. And if I didn't get enough sleep, my work the next day would suffer, because the fact of it was, I was still *learning* what it was that I needed to do at work. I needed to sleep, and since I was exclusively breastfeeding, it was a little difficult to catch a break. There was no "it's Daddy's turn to heat up the bottle," like in those old sitcoms with the beleaguered dad standing by the stove with a bottle in a saucepan (invariably, the dad is wearing blue-striped pajamas)—when Cal needed to eat, it was always me who had to get up.

Furthermore, and perhaps more to the point, I find that I really miss my baby. It is the first year of my Anesthesia residency, and I am working a lot. These early months, with Cal so young, I might come home from work and see him for an hour or two before it's time for him to go to bed. There are some nights where, apart from bedtime, Joe or I will barely see Cal at all. And the idea of spending fourteen hours a day away from our baby, only to deliberately sequester him in another room for another eight hours while we are actually home and he clearly wants to be close to us...well, that just doesn't feel good to us. In fact, it feels bad.

And so it ends up that Cal is cosleeping with us. We clear a space for him between the two of us on our queen-sized mattress, make sure the pillows and blankets are away from his face, and there we are, a family of three, there in the bed. Anytime we want to see him at night, touch him, smell his little peach-fuzz head, there he is. Anytime he needs us, is hungry, cold, there we are. And everyone gets to sleep. Perhaps it is an imperfect system, and we might not be doing it if we had more time to spend with him during our waking hours, but this is what works for us, so that is what we are doing.

I will not concede on the vaccinations, though. Any kid of mine is going to get vaccinated. I am still, after all, a doctor, and my crunchy-granola-mom inclinations will take me only so far.

* * *

It is now January of my first year of residency, and for better or for worse, we have adjusted to being a two-resident household with a baby. Since Cal was born, I have new routines at work, new habits that are built into my routine. For instance, now it is 1:36 p.m., and I am eating a pepperoni pizza Hot Pocket in the shower stall of the women's locker room, two plastic cones pushed down my bra, the tubing to the breast pump dangling between my knees.

Of course, to call my lunch a "Hot Pocket" is not totally precise. That is the brand name, of course, but I didn't actually heat it up, because I don't have time. Usually I allot myself five minutes out of my thirty-minute lunch break to the process of retrieving and heating my food, but today, a nurse who was a little quicker than I reached the microwave first and started rewarming her leftovers from the night before—some sort of overpoweringly pungent fish stew. I look at the indicator on the microwave: *three minutes, fifty-eight seconds left*. I do not have an additional three minutes and fifty-eight seconds. So I will eat my Hot Pocket cold.

The shower stall in which I sit to eat my lunch every day is another concession to necessity. There is—and it seems almost foolish to expect otherwise—no lactation suite in the adult hospital. Nor is there a private room within ready reach of the OR with both a door and an electrical socket. There *are* actually a few lactation rooms over by the Neonatal ICU in the Children's Hospital, equipped with locking doors and sinks and even a few chairs—these are rooms for patients, of course, or new mothers with babies in the NICU, though employees sometimes use these rooms too if they're not occupied. But given that it would take ten minutes to walk over from the ORs to the NICU and ten minutes to walk back, these lactation rooms might as well be in Brooklyn.

I have tried on several occasions to pump elsewhere. One good spot I found was in the patient changing rooms over at the Cystoscopy suite, which, while not immediately adjacent to the operating rooms, were close enough. I was friendly with the nurses who worked there, and while they never asked what exactly I was doing back there and I never told them, their conspiratorial winks led me to believe that they knew. There were two changing rooms in the back with curtains that could be drawn closed, and one of the changing rooms even had an outlet I could plug my pump into. There was no room for a chair, but I didn't mind sitting on the floor. It was well lit and convenient enough, though the preponderance of half-nude old men wandering in and out of the area demanding to know "where in the hell that noise is coming from" gradually made me stop going there. So instead, I hide out each day in the shower stall.

The showers in the locker room have long since stopped working—the room is now used for storage

of maintenance equipment, and some of the staff
sometimes hang their winter coats over the shower
rods when their lockers are overstuffed. It is a dim
room—you would need a penlight to read fine print
in there—made all the more gloomy by the fact that
one of the overhead fixtures always seems to be broken. There is always something a little unsavory in
there—a stash of soiled linens, a bucket with a moist
mop, some sort of dusty OR equipment from back in
the days of anesthesia-free amputations—but there is
an outlet and a chair and the shower curtain at least
offers some degree of mildewed, grimy privacy.

I have rigged my breast pump to be a hands-free
device, so while I eat my Cold Pocket with one hand,
I am on the phone with the other, conferring with
our nanny. Cal, now six months old, had a fever last
night, and I am calling to check in. After asking a
few more questions and reconfirming the Tylenol-
dosing schedule should the need come up, I hang up
and place a call to my pediatrician's office. I am under
no impression that Cal needs to see a doctor for this
fever—as a former Pediatrics resident in the trenches
myself, I know that even the best-intentioned doctors
are basically useless for this kind of run-of-the-mill
viral scourge—but Cal needs an appointment for his
six-month checkup, and as usual I am late in getting
him in to be seen. I am put on hold mid-greeting by
the harried receptionist, and after waiting for what
feels like an eternity (though my watch confirms that
it was only one minute and thirty-eight seconds),
I land an appointment for six weeks from now, on
one of my post-call days off. The appointment is for

9:30 a.m.—I will have just enough time to get home, shower, change, and get Cal ready before jumping on the subway uptown. I tell the receptionist that I will take the appointment time and hang up.

It is 1:52 and I need to hustle. Quickly, I bottle up the milk, giving the used equipment a perfunctory rinse (as if life was not complicated enough, there have been trace amounts of *Legionella* bacteria found in the hospital water supply, so I bring my own rinse water from home in a thermos), and hurriedly bag everything back up again. I run to the refrigerator, stick the contents of my insulated cooler inside, toward the back. Then, with two minutes left to spare, I put my surgical mask back on and run back into the OR, where my neurosurgical case, a craniotomy to remove a brain tumor, is still proceeding apace. The attending who has been taking care of the patient during my lunch break looks up from his laptop and gives me a quick update before leaving the room.

The one thing that I actually *didn't* get to do on my lunch break—the one thing that I probably *needed* to do—was use the bathroom. But it is too late now, and I'm certainly not going to ask my attending for an extra ninety seconds. There are another two-and-a-half hours left to go in the surgery, and I can certainly cross my legs until then. The last thing I want to do in my situation, as a resident who had the temerity to take a maternity leave, is appear like I am asking for any special treatment for any reason. I do not want to be treated any differently than any other resident, lest people resent me for "playing the baby card" and currying special favor. In fact, I make an effort to overcompensate—showing up extra early in the mornings, rarely taking the full time off during my breaks, making it a point to never, ever complain. I do not want to appear weak, because as a female resident with an infant at home, I feel almost like people are expecting me to be. In fact, unless someone specifically asks, I usually try not to bring up the fact that I have a baby at all. It just seems easier that way.

I am on call again, and later that same evening, I am dealing with an emergency case in the operating room, an elderly man who broke his hip two days ago after he slipped walking down the steps in front of his house. I administer a spinal anesthetic to numb the surgical site, the spinal needle slipping between his vertebrae, with that disconcerting feeling of bouncing off arthritic bone and crunchy, calcified ligaments. Luckily, we find the sweet spot and our spinal sets up well, and with the sedative infusion running in through his IV the patient is snoring comfortably. Fatigued, I gaze at his vitals on the monitor, my mind wandering a little bit, until I look down with a start—my hip is vibrating. I have just been paged, and, alarmingly, my home phone number shows up on the display. You know that feeling of dread you get when your phone rings at 2:00 a.m.? That feeling of, "Who died?" This is the feeling I get every time I get paged to my own home.

"Hello?" I whisper into the receiver. Joe has picked up. I can hear Cal crying in the background.

"Hello?" Joe raises his voice to be heard over the squalling. "Where are you? I can barely hear you."

"I'm . . ." I pause as the orthopedic surgeon picks up a drill and, with a little test *whirr*, drives a screw squealing into my patient's femur. "I'm in the OR."

"I can't hear you. Why are you talking so quietly?"

It seems too much effort to explain the picture, and the fact that I don't want the surgeons to hear that I am making a personal call on the OR phone. "I'm in the OR," I say again, a little louder, lifting up my mask so that my voice is not as muffled. "What's going on? Is Cal OK?"

"He's fine," Joe tells me. But he then goes on to say, "He still has a little fever, though. I just took his temperature. 103.4 rectally." He pauses. "He's a little fussy, I guess."

"Table up, please," Brian, the ortho resident, booms. He is the classic orthopedic surgeon, one of those exceedingly large and well-muscled men for whom the concept of speaking quietly is completely foreign. Giving him a *you got it* thumbs-up, I stretch the phone cord to its limit until I can reach the bed controls and move the patient up about an inch. "Good," he intones, and goes back at it.

I turn my attention back to the phone. "How does he look, though? Does he have a rash? Is he drinking? How have his diapers been today? Is he making good urine?" I am asking the questions rapid-fire now, the way that I would during my nights in the trenches of the Peds ER. In my mind, I am already cycling through worst-case scenarios. *Febrile seizure. Inability to tolerate fluids requiring hospitalization for IV hydration. Sepsis secondary to some strain of*

*hospital-cultivated, multi-antibiotic resistant bacte-
ria that Joe or I brought home with us.* Like many
of the type A personalities in medicine, I have been a
fairly neurotic person my whole life, but not until Cal
was born did I realize just how *much* I had to worry
about.

"No rash, he's drinking OK, diapers have been
OK. I think he's just a little pokey because of his temp
being so high. I'm going to give him some Tylenol."

"OK. You know the dosing, right? Ten to fifteen
milligrams per kilogram?" I pronounce this last *migs
per kig*, the shorthand from the wards, like waitresses
at diners calling for "Adam and Eve on a raft, burn
'em." "Cal weighs about seventeen pounds, that's 7.7
kigs." I am tapping on my calculator now, doing this
conversion by reflex, as in my days on Pediatrics.
"That'll be around 115 migs, Children's Tylenol is
160 migs per teaspoon, so you'll want to give him"—
I double-check my math—"3.5 mils. Just make sure
you're giving him the Children's Tylenol, though,
not the Infant's Tylenol with the dropper, because the
infant elixir is much more concentrated, 80 migs per
mil, so...you know."

Joe is checking the math himself. "Yeah, that looks
right. I'll mix it in with some applesauce or something, see if he'll take it."

"He can get dosed every four hours," I remind Joe,
though I know he knows as well as I do. "Call me
if he starts getting a rash or if he's not taking fluids or—" I think of all the things I want to say right
now, and a five-minute phone conversation seems insufficient to convey the full extent of guilt and worry

that I am feeling, working overnight in the hospital while my baby is sick at home—"*anything.* You can call me anytime. Or page me. E-mail me an update before you go to sleep, if you get a chance."

I hang up the phone and step back toward the OR table, where the surgeons have placed the screw satisfactorily and are taking multiple shots with the portable X-ray machine to make sure everything is aligned and in place. I look down at my patient, feeling distracted and detached, and wonder to myself, *Why am I here? Why am I taking care of* you, *a person I've never even* met *until half an hour ago, a stranger, while my own child is sick at home and needs his mother? I've been away from him for sixteen hours and it will be at least another twelve before I see him again—what am I doing? Why, when my own family needs me, am I taking care of* you? And then I snap back to my surroundings at the head of the table, see the liver-spotted pate barely covered by a few wispy strands of nicotine-stained white hair, think of this old man, living alone, slipping and falling in front of his house as he hazarded the brutal winter weather to go out for groceries. And I feel ashamed of my earlier thoughts. I'm a doctor. This is *exactly* who I should be taking care of.

"How's she doing?" asks Brian, who by this time has not only completely forgotten the patient's name, but also the fact that the "she" is a man, despite the fact that he is drilling only six inches away from the patient's groin.

"The patient is fine." And he is, still sleeping comfortably, snoring slightly, all his vitals stable up on the screen. I put my hand gently on the patient's forehead. "He's going to be fine."

Nights

Certain things in the hospital seem to happen only at night. Babies, for example, always seem to be born at night, as though they've timed it for maximal inconvenience. Certain emergency surgeries, like appendectomies, surgeries for ectopic pregnancy, and organ transplants, also always seem to go at night. On the flip side of this, there is another surgery that is almost always scheduled after hours. This surgery is more of an urgency than an emergency, is of no benefit to the patient himself, but it is as rigorously choreographed as anything else that happens in the hospital.

It is early winter during my first year as an anesthesia resident when I am called to staff an organ harvest.

The patient is a middle-aged man currently housed in the Neurosurgical Intensive Care Unit who suffered a massive bleed in his brain several days ago, probably resulting from the rupture of an aneurysm he never even knew he had. He was intubated by EMS on the scene, brought to the hospital, and declared brain-dead yesterday afternoon. His family, upon consultation with the transplant team, has agreed to donate his kidneys.

"What, *just* his kidneys?" is the first question I ask, setting up the operating room, drawing up the necessary meds and making sure my anesthesia machine is up and running. "What's wrong with his other organs?" The nurse assigned to scrub for the case shrugs, and tells me that sometimes families have some sort of ideological hang-ups about donating specific organs, especially the heart or the eyes. I can understand this, I guess, but in a young, reasonably healthy man, to donate one pair of organs and not the others seems like such a waste.

"It's weird that they call it an 'organ harvest,' don't you think?" I am still talking to the nurse, who is busy setting up things on her end. "It's like..." and I pantomime plucking fruit and putting it into a basket. "Why do they call it that, do you suppose? Does it sound better than saying *organ collection* or *organ retrieval*, like it gives families less of this impression that we're, like, killing people to steal their corneas or whatever?"

"I don't know," the nurse replies, "all I know is after I saw my first organ harvest, I crossed out that organ donation box on the back of my driver's license."

"Meaning you decided to donate your organs?"

"No," she corrects me, "I decided *not* to donate my organs."

I am confused. "But why? Because I've done anesthesia for these kidney transplant recipients, and they're just so happy when their number comes up. You know, they're, like, crying with joy and everything."

"Yeah. Maybe I should change it back. But the first harvest I saw kind of turned me off. I didn't like how it was at the end."

"What do you mean?" I ask. I've never done a harvest before and am curious.

"Well, the last harvest I did, it was a really young guy, and they took everything. Heart, liver, pancreas, *everything*. There were, like, twenty-odd people in the room. And after they all got what they wanted, everyone left, and the patient was just lying here, alone. I peeked behind the curtain to look for Anesthesia, and *they* were gone, too. Everyone was gone except for me and the patient. And it kind of left a bad impression."

"Oh." I think about this. "That *does* sound pretty bad."

I pause, considering this. I think back to one patient in particular I took care of for her kidney transplant, a middle-aged woman who had been on dialysis for more than two years before she finally got a donor match. *This is my second chance,* she told me prior to being wheeled into the operating room, the joy and relief beaming from her face as clearly as any image projected on a screen in our old med school lecture hall.

"You *should* check that box off though. On your license, I mean," I say. Trying to inject some levity into the discussion, I continue, "I would treat you real nice if I had to do your harvest."

The nurse turns to me, considering. "Yeah, you know, maybe I will someday."

Hastily, realizing what I just said, I add, "Hopefully it never comes up, though. Hopefully you'll be so old and gnarled when you die that we won't want to touch your organs with a ten-foot pole."

She laughs. "Yeah, I hope so too."

An hour later, the patient is wheeled down from the ICU, and we move him onto the operating table. He doesn't *look* dead. He's warm, his skin is soft and pink, his chest moving up and down on the ventilator just like all the other patients I take care of. On the monitors, his vital signs are picture perfect, like out of a textbook. I've had patients who were technically more alive than him look much worse.

"Turn on some gas and give him a little fentanyl," my senior resident instructs me prior to incision. Before I can ask him why, he responds, "He can't *feel* anything, obviously, but he may still have a sympathetic response to surgery, and we want to keep his pressure down to protect the organs before they cross-clamp." He means that the more primitive pathways of the nervous system may still be active, and though the patient is technically brain-dead and unable to feel pain, his body may still respond to surgical insult by jacking up his heart rate and blood pressure, which could damage his kidneys prior to harvest.

The incision is different from those that I've seen in other surgeries. For other patients, the cuts are small and low, to minimize postsurgical scarring and to create a better cosmetic effect. In this patient, however, the incision is "stem to stern," a huge vertical incision straight down the entire abdomen, from the tip of the xyphoid process at the base of the sternum down to the top of the patient's pubic bone. The size of the incision in this case is for the benefit of the surgeons procuring the organs, not for the benefit of the patient himself.

219

Because he's dead, I keep having to remind my-self. *This patient is dead.*

The retrieval proceeds quickly, the surgeons dissecting briskly through the different layers of fat and muscle until the kidneys on both sides are laid bare. Then clamps are applied, isolating the blood flow to the organs, and then both kidneys are liberated from the patient's body. In a sense, the kidneys *are* the patient now—all the attention from the entire OR team has turned to tending to the organs, which warrant their own ID bands and paperwork. The surgeons handle them tenderly, bathing them in an ice bath and packing them up in preparation to join the next body requiring their service. The actual patient who still lies on the OR table, abdomen held open by retractors but with no salvageable organs left, is apparently not necessary anymore.

"OK, they're out, so turn off the vent," my senior resident instructs with a casual air. I know he has never done an organ harvest either—he told me so himself before starting the surgery—so I'm surprised at how cavalier he is about this, how bizarre it feels to be in this role.

"Just...you know...turn it *off*?" I know what he's telling me, and what I have to do, but am just trying to buy myself time. Intellectually it makes sense to me, but after working all day to keep patients alive, being the one who actually turns *off* life support feels like fifteen shades of wrong.

"Yeah, he's already been declared brain-dead, remember? Just turn it off, and we're done." I peek over the drape into the surgical field. Already, the surgeons are closing up the incision. Not the transplant surgeons who did the actual harvest—they're long gone—but a junior resident, who is closing not with small meticulous stitches in multiple layers to facilitate a tight closure and healing, but with a length of thick suture on a large needle, going through all the layers of skin and fat and muscle in one large swipe. I've seen closures like this before, in the morgue after an autopsy.

Following orders, I reach over to my machine, flip the switch, and the ventilator is off. The patient's chest stops moving. Over the next few minutes, I stand and watch as the measured oxygen saturation of the blood starts drifting down. Alarms sound, and I turn them off. The heart begins to slow and then to fibrillate. It takes everything I have not to reach over, turn the ventilator back on, start resuscitating, to *do* something. To stand by and watch as these vital signs deteriorate seems as unnatural as—well, as looking at this warm, pink patient and calling him a dead man.

My senior resident is already walking out the door—besides us, the only people left in the room are the surgical resident, putting in his last few stitches, and the circulating nurse, who is already preparing the body bag. As the anesthesiologists, our job here is finished. "Come on, we've got other stuff to do. Grab your bag." And he exits the OR, not looking back to see if I'm following.

I would like to say that I stayed. That would have been a better ending to this story. I would like to say that despite the fact that the patient was dead, and that there was no real good reason for me to be there, that I stayed anyway. To help get the body ready. To take out all our invasive equipment. Out of respect for the patient, who through his death was now going to save someone else, and who, though dead, was *still* my patient. I should have stayed, but I was expected not to, and so I did not. I still regret it.

* * *

It is 1:00 a.m. in the Surgical Intensive Care Unit, and I am starving.

Apparently everyone else in the ICU is too, because the refrigerator is empty. There is a small, dorm-sized fridge under the ice machine in one of the small alcoves off the nursing station, which is supposed to be stocked with food for the patients. But in this unit, hardly any of the patients are well enough to eat, and the food ends up being consumed mostly by the staff. There is nothing *good* in there, mind you, but there is hospital food that is technically edible. Jell-O cups, saltine crackers, cans of off-brand ginger ale, occasionally small shrink-wrapped packets of processed cheese. Any of these will do in a pinch.

I go through the emptied cupboards of the pantry looking for something, *anything*, that I might have missed. A small pack of graham crackers that fell behind the shelf, perhaps. Or a small foil-topped cup of juice. But all I can locate are cans of calorie-dense liquid nutritional supplements for our tube-fed patients. *What does Jevity taste like?* I wonder, considering the can. *I mean, they probably don't make any special effort to have it taste good, since it usu-*

ally bypasses the taste buds entirely, but maybe...on ice...it might not be half-bad?

A nurse pokes her head around the corner to interrupt my hypoglycemic reverie. "Room Nine expired. You need to come and call it." And then she's gone, walking briskly back down the hall, hunter green scrubs swishing. This, apparently, is the preferred terminology in the ICU. Patients do not "die" or "pass away" here, rather they *expire*, like a carton of milk in the back of the dairy section.

"Thank you, I'll be right there," I call. After looking at the can of Jevity one more time and conceding that when an information label reads, *"may be used for oral feeding of patients with altered taste perception,"* it means that the stuff probably tastes like shit, I place it back on the shelf and follow the nurse into the patient's room.

There have been no surprises in Room 9 that night. Mrs. Altagracia Tavares has been with us in the ICU for weeks, having barely survived two liver transplants in the past few months, and despite all our best efforts, she is critically, terminally ill. The decision had been made in a big family meeting with the ICU team, the transplant surgeons, and the Tavares family a few days ago that Mrs. Tavares will be made DNR (Do Not Resuscitate). We will withdraw most of the more heroic measures keeping her alive, including hemodialysis (she has long since gone into kidney failure), and we will not escalate any of the medications maintaining her blood pressure or her heart function. Instead, we will leave her on the ventilator, allow nature to take its course, letting her die if not in peace, then at least without the orchestrated violence of an active resuscitation involving chest compression and shocks with the defibrillator that would not, in all likelihood, change the outcome. "She'll probably go tonight," her primary resident told me upon signing out earlier this evening. It had been two days since we had withdrawn dialysis. Her vital signs have been spiraling downward. And now, as we expected, she is dead.

I approach the room, respectful of the family that has gathered together this evening in anticipation of their matriarch's passing. I suddenly remember an embarrassing mark on the back of my white coat—earlier, I accidentally sat in a puddle of spilled coffee that has since dried into an unsightly yellowish stain, making it look like I peed on myself—and angle myself slightly away from the family before anyone can see. The patient's EKG is tracing a flatline on the screen, and I indicate to the nurse to turn off all the monitors still tethered to the patient's body, sparing her husband and her sons the further trauma of seeing the alarms, the flashing warnings that a heart rate of zero is *not* a good thing. I listen intently to her chest with my stethoscope though already knowing what I will find. Nothing. I feel her carotid for a pulse. Nothing. I look at her pupils, shine a light to assess their responsiveness, and see no reaction from those vast, black circles. "We can turn off the vent." I indicate to the nurse, and the ventilator powers off with a brief, protesting wail. "Time of death"—I look at my watch—"one twelve."

And that, as they say, is the ball game. It *should* be. But it is not.

Mrs. Tavares makes a sudden, convulsive movement, opening her mouth with a sudden intake of breath like a fish gasping on a dock. The family, who had finally become comfortable with the idea that their mother is at peace, pauses and looks at me questioningly. "Agonal breathing," I reassure them. "A reflex. Sometimes, after a patient's heart stops, it happens. She's comfortable. She's not in pain." The family members nod, look reassured, and file out to tell the rest of the assembled clan in the waiting area that the vigil is over. I continue to stay at the bedside with the nurse, watching the patient. Thirty seconds later, the patient gasps again. Twenty seconds after that, again. We keep watching and waiting for her to stop. Altagracia Tavares refuses to comply.

"I'm just going to call admitting and let them know that we have a patient who just expired," I tell the nurse. Declaring patients dead is a bureaucratic business, involving filing a report with the medical examiner's office and getting the death certificate printed for my signature. The sooner I get things rolling, I figure, the better. I spend some time on the phone taking care of this unpleasantness. I return to Mrs. Tavares's room five minutes later, walking in while she is in mid-gasp.

"*Still* at it?" I am starting to feel uncomfortable. How long is she supposed to keep this up? The fact of it is that I have not declared very many people dead before, and those that I *have* declared had the good sense to lie down and *act* dead, not create a scene like

225

the one that is unfolding right here. "She *was* asystolic when you called me in here, right?" I ask the nurse. "I mean, before we turned the monitors off?" The nurse nods, confirming that the patient had gone into ventricular fibrillation shortly before 1:00 a.m., after which point she became asystolic, a flatline tracing on her EKG. "OK, just checking. I mean, not that you don't know what you're doing, and not like we would have done anything about it *anyway*, because, you know..." I indicate the DNR order. Altagracia Tavares gasps again. It has now been ten minutes since I declared her dead.

"I know she's dead," I say, feeling less and less sure of myself, "but...could we just flip the monitors back on for a second? I just want to see." The monitors come back on, and as we expected, the EKG is tracing a flatline. *Flatline, flatline, flatline.* And then, one little irregular blip. Many more seconds pass. Flatline. Then another blip. And then—I really can't believe what I am seeing now—more and more beats, until Mrs. Tavares is back up to an irregular heart rate of about 50. "It's probably just PEA," I say, ostensibly to the nurse but mostly to myself—that is, pulseless electrical activity, lines on an EKG without a heartbeat—still nothing we would interfere with, since the patient's family explicitly wants no resuscitation, no new cardioactive drugs. But to confirm, I go to feel for a pulse.

There is a pulse.

"Holy crap," I say, "she's *back*." Peeking outside to make sure that the patient's family is well down the hallway, out of earshot, I start, discreetly, to lose my shit. "Have you ever *seen* someone be asystolic for, like, *ten minutes,* and then get a pulse back? What the hell *is* this?"

"Sometimes it happens," says the nurse, quite blasé, probably because she has seen literally hundreds more people die than I have. "What do you want to do?"

"She has a pulse, so we *have* to put her back on the vent, right? Her family didn't want ventilatory support withdrawn before she died, and now she's sort of technically not *dead* anymore, so I think we have to turn it back on. I mean, her heart will stop again later on, and we can turn the vent off again then, but if she has a *pulse,* I think we're kind of obligated to, you know, *ventilate* her, right? Right?" I am now completely out of my comfort zone, in the resident's worst-case scenario of It's Life and Death and I Don't Know What the Hell I'm Doing. I mean, what do you do when you declare a patient Dead and then, ten minutes later, they decide to become Not Dead?

So with another flip of the switch, we put Mrs. Tavares back on the vent, and after making sure that the settings are correct, I go out to the nursing station to call Oliver, the critical care fellow overseeing the ICU overnight. "Wait, why did you turn the monitors back on?" Oliver asks first thing, halfway through my admittedly convoluted story.

"She fucking got a *pulse* back, dude!" I splutter. Oliver comes down a few minutes later, surveys the scene, and exits the room shaking his head and muttering something in German. He says he can't make heads or tails of it either, but that I should just stay the course and call him when she inevitably dies again. *Oh, like it's that easy,* I want to say.

I call back the admitting office to tell them to hold off on that death certificate for now. Then I go talk to the family. This is probably the hardest part, because I don't really know what to *say.* I do think they understand that Altagracia is, for all intents and purposes, *dead,* as people with no blood flow to the brain for ten minutes will be, but from the expressions on their faces, I can see that they are definitely confused by the whole heartbeat-no-heartbeat-oh-wait-yes-there's-a-heartbeat thing. *Join the club,* I think, though thankfully, I do not say this aloud. Instead, I excuse myself, return to the ICU, and settle myself in for the wait.

A few hours later, as the sun is coming up, Mrs. Tavares "expires" again. This time around, I touch nothing. "Let's wait another few minutes, just to be sure," I tell the nurse, gun-shy from before. But this time her heart stays silent. She has no pulse, her pupils do not react, she does not blink when I press a small fluff of cotton swab to her cornea. After about fifteen minutes, we turn off the monitors and take her off the vent for the last time.

There are some lessons learned in residency that are clear, and some that are not. I would *like* to say that my experience with Altagracia Tavares taught me something profound about life and death, about medical futility and ethics. After treading for a few hours on that razor-thin line separating death and not-death, I would like to have come away having learned something huge and lasting. But to be honest, the lesson I came away with after that night was this: if someone's dead and you *know* they're dead, perhaps the best and most humane thing to do is to turn off those monitors and just keep them off.

* * *

Almost nine months into working parenthood, Joe and I are relatively mechanized in our daily routine. For instance, our call schedules. I am on call about twice a week, and Joe sometimes more than that, and we have managed to work it out such that we never take call on the same night. We make call requests in advance, trade call nights with our classmates, take extra call during each other's days off, whatever it takes so that one of us can be home with the baby every evening. Of course, this method is not perfect—medicine is not always predictable, and often we find ourselves working later than expected even on nights that we are not officially scheduled to—but we are managing.

The same goes for weekends. We try to offset which weekends either of us have to be at work, so that at least one of us can be home with the baby. Occasionally, we will even *both* have the same weekend off, which we try to spend doing some sort of family activity (grocery shopping counts), but for the most part, the most difficult part about having a baby is that Joe and I feel like we rarely see each other. It's like being on "night float" all over again.

Despite our intricate scheduling system, all coordinated by a four-color-coded paper calendar hanging in the kitchen (increasingly tattered from all the handling), there is one catastrophic event for which we have no failsafe. Our entire weekly schedule, our entire day-to-day existence, hinges on the fact that we have childcare, and that while Joe and I go to work, there is someone to stay home with Cal.

Then, in the spring of my first year of Anesthesia residency, we fire our nanny.

It pains me to admit it, but there were signs early on our nanny—the one we inherited with such good references—was not a good fit. Troublesome interactions, unreasonable demands, the number of times this past year that I came home to find Cal floundering in his playpen surrounded by dust bunnies while she sat on the couch, laughing at the antics of that ever-delightful Damon Wayans on *My Wife and Kids*. I know these are long hours we're all working, and that everyone needs a break once in a while, but it was concerning that not only did she not look up when the baby was crying, she hardly even looked up when *I* came home.

But for months I looked the other way. I made excuses for her, provided suggestions so gentle they probably didn't even register, and forgave her all but the most glaring transgressions, because—why? Because it felt awkward and classist to be someone's boss, especially when that person was older than you? Because I wanted her to like me? Because I didn't want her to be upset? Because she spent more time with my son than I did, and the last thing I wanted to do was offend her in some way?

Or (and this is probably as close to the truth as I can

get) because given our circumstances, we didn't think that we *could* do any better than this, doubted that we would be able to find another nanny to work these hours—and quite frankly, we *needed* her, flaws and all, so that Joe and I could go to work every day. If we fired her, or if she quit, we would not be able to leave the house every morning, so that we could take care of our patients while she took care of our child. *She needs to stay so that we can leave.* And so I *needed* to pretend that she was doing a good job, because otherwise, how could I function? How could I willingly leave the house every morning knowing that Cal would be doing better staying at home with me? If I allowed myself to see this truth, think these thoughts, I would never be able to walk out the door every morning. So for the sake of my career, I pretend. I looked on the bright side ("She's very experienced! The family she was with before just could not say enough good things about her!"), turned a blind eye to her problems, and praised her lavishly to anyone who asked, though I'm not sure who, exactly, I was trying to convince.

I'm not sure how much longer I would have put off the inevitable had our nanny herself not brought the issue to a head. Out of nowhere early in the spring, she demands a huge raise ahead of schedule, and despite being told that 50 percent of the net income of our household is already being diverted directly into her pocket (we actually show her our paystubs from the hospital), negotiations escalate and become acrimonious on her end, to the point that, after that evening, we decide that she will not be in our employ any longer.

I will never forget the lessons that we learn from this, our first experience with full-time childcare. First is that regardless of who is employing whom, any set of parents with full-time, inflexible jobs are essentially held hostage by those who are taking care of their children during the day. And the second is that despite our two incomes, our most financially advantageous move at this point and probably most beneficial for the baby would be if either Joe or I quit residency and stayed home full-time.

"You could always quit if you wanted, I would support that decision if that's what you wanted," Joe has said more than once even before this juncture, usually after some period of grumbling and idle threats on my part to do just that. And I have offered the same support to him, though, as The Man, he takes that suggestion even less seriously than I do. The problem with combining medical training with parenthood is that neither deserves anything less than your full attention, and to attempt to do both simultaneously is to feel that you are doing neither well. A negligent doctor by day, a half-assed parent by night. The option to concentrate on just *one* of those vocations occasionally becomes tempting, an ever-present escape hatch that we keep eyeing. *I could quit,* I think occasionally, during those late nights or long days away from home. *What's more important to me, my family or my job? Is this really worth it? Am I missing my son's entire childhood, allowing him to be raised by other people? What could justify that? What could possibly make all this worth it?*

I tell myself these things to give myself the possibility of an out, but really, I never seriously consider leaving medicine. It's not just the years I've already invested in training or the hundreds of thousands of dollars I've spent on tuition. It's not just the rationalization that babies grow up, go to school, grow into their own, separate lives, and that when that happens, I need a separate life too. It's not even the love of practicing medicine—that is, while I do *enjoy* my vocation, I rarely wake up for work whooping with glee, a laryngoscope already in one hand and a central line kit in the other. Rather, it's the notion, so ingrained in the culture of medicine that it is almost never explicitly stated: that just because something is *hard* is no reason not to do it; that in fact, there are few things worth doing that don't require significant sacrifice along the way.

But these are lofty issues, a conversation that deserves a nice dinner and a glass of wine and that can be discussed at a later date. The issue now, *right now*, is how, freshly nannyless, Joe and I are going to be able to go to work tomorrow morning.

"Should one of us take a day off tomorrow, you think? Stay home with the baby?"

"Take a day off from residency. You're funny. Did anyone ever tell you that you're funny?"

It is, of course, strongly discouraged for residents to take personal days or call in sick, even if they are, you know, *actually sick*. In fact, one of the orthopedic residents, sick with the flu, had just completed a total knee replacement the other day, turning away from the patient and lifting his mask to vomit into one of the OR garbage cans—though only after completing the final skin stitch, a fact that he conveyed with some pride. One anesthesia attending once told me point blank that there is never any excuse for a resident to call in sick. "If you're not sick enough to be hospitalized," he reasoned, "you should be at work. And if you *are* sick enough to be hospitalized, *you work at a hospital.* What better place to be?" So obviously, the idea of missing work for a babysitting issue is even more unthinkable. But with a nine-month-old baby and no childcare, what alternative do we have? What else would we do? Bring Cal to work with us? Put a little surgical mask on him, wrap him in sterile drapes, and prop him up in the corner?

Luckily, we have some options. My parents, alerted to the situation, promptly rearrange their own work schedules—my father cancels all his clinic patients for the morning, and my mother all her patients for the afternoon. And thus they trade off childcare for the next four days, alternating shifts, until we eventually find a new nanny at the end of the week. When I timidly put forth the offer for either Joe or me to take a day off to share the load, my father dismisses this notion as ridiculous. "Take a day off during residency? Because you don't have a *babysitter*? Don't be insane. Your mother and I are attendings now. We can rearrange our schedules. But you and Joe are residents, so you can't. Don't even consider it. Just go to work."

In recent years there has been no shortage of magazine or Internet articles touting the success of the new face of working motherhood, each showcasing a handful of such modern "mommies" (a cutesy designation which sets my teeth on edge) who, through varying degrees of sacrifice and negotiation, are able to "have it all." Eager for hints, or at least some degree of absolution from reading about other working mothers feeling equally strapped and harried, I never fail to head straight for these articles, only to find the same unhelpful pointers every time. *Work flextime!* the articles invariably suggest. *Pick a day or two a week to work from home! Take a leave of absence! If the company you're with doesn't offer you the flexibility you need, consider starting your own business!* Who *are* these people? Where do they work? What *planet* do they live on where these things are even a possibility?

The message I get from society is clear: the ability to juggle working motherhood successfully is contingent upon having the right *kind* of job. And medical residency is clearly the absolute wrongest kind of job you could have—inflexible within a historically patriarchal system, where sacrifice of one's personal life toward the service of others is part of the ingrained and expected. All the messages we get from the establishment on both sides tell us this loud and clear: *You can have your medical career, or you can be a good parent. The sooner you realize this, the happier you will be.*

And, you know, on some level, the naysayers are probably right. Probably it's *not* really reasonable to expect to "have it all." There are only so many hours in the day, after all, and too many things competing for your attention during those hours. You cannot do everything, be everywhere, and take care of yourself all at once. It's simply not possible.

But that doesn't stop us from trying.

* * *

It is now my second year of Anesthesia residency, and I am rotating through the ICU again, only this time, instead of the Surgical Intensive Care Unit (or the SICU, which we residents pronounce "the sick-you" with complete lack of irony), I am in the Cardiothoracic Intensive Care Unit, or CTICU. Whereas the SICU manages a wide range of postsurgical patients requiring care in a more monitored setting—meaning patients on vasoactive drips and ventilators, septic and comatose after surgeries ranging from Cesarean sections to liver transplants—the CTICU is specifically designated for patients after open-heart or lung surgery. The nurses are specially trained in the care of these patients, the cardiac and thoracic surgeons make rounds here in the morning, and we Anesthesia residents have the experience of rotating through after our month doing cardiothoracic anesthesia in the operating rooms. Basically, this allows us to see what becomes of our open-heart patients after they leave our ORs.

I am the overnight resident on call in the CTICU tonight, and so far the night is shaping up to be—dare I say it—not too bad. My patients are sick, of course, and any patient in the ICU is potentially on the brink of spontaneously doing something floridly horrible, but on the whole, no one is misbehaving. I walk by the bed of one post–heart transplant patient and relish the muttered snoring I hear issuing forth from the semidarkened room. Not only does this noise mean that the patient is extubated, it means he is actually *sleeping*. Glancing quickly at his monitors, I hope that nothing happens for the rest of the night that requires me to wake him up.

At around 11:00 p.m., one more admission rolls into Room 1, taking the last empty bed in the unit. The patient, Anne Brennan, is a ninety-year-old woman coming up from a late case in the cardiac catheterization lab, having just had a percutaneous replacement of a leaking aortic valve. The traditional aortic valve replacement is an open-heart procedure that involves bringing the patient to the OR, sawing open their sternum, and putting them on a heart lung machine, with a potentially prolonged recovery in the CTICU afterward. In contrast, a percutaneous valve replacement gains access to the heart through the femoral artery, snaking a catheter up into the aorta and above the patient's native aortic valve, where an artificial valve is deployed and anchored in place. It is still a relatively new procedure, with complication rates to match the learning curve, but it seems to be a viable alternative, and obviously much less invasive for the patients. Though I have seen patients with catastrophic outcomes and mortal complications after percutaneous valve replacements, my new patient seems to be doing swimmingly. Her vital signs are stable, her skin is warm and pink, she is extubated and talking soon after her procedure, even joking with me and her nurse with a voice that still holds a trace of an Irish accent. *Swish.* It's 2:30 a.m. in the CTICU and we're having a good night.

About forty-five minutes later, I am called into Ms. Brennan's room by her nurse, Angel. "I just wanted to show you this," he says, and lifts up the thin white sheet covering Ms. Brennan's legs. Up high on her left thigh, in the crease where leg meets pelvis and spreading underneath the small dressing covering the puncture site where the surgeons obtained femoral artery access, is a coaster-sized purplish bruise.

"Is everything all right?" Ms. Brennan asks politely. Even at this hour, her accent sounds adorably like something out of an Irish Spring commercial, one of the old ones where they slice through the edge of the soap with a pocketknife, presumably to show how pure and clean it is.

"Everything's fine," I tell her. "You just have a little bruising from where they put in the catheter. It's not uncommon, but we're going to keep an eye on it, OK?" Gesturing to Angel discreetly, I pull him aside and ask in a quieter voice, "How did it look when she came up here?"

"A little bruised, but I think it's getting bigger. Kind of hard to say."

"Well, let's monitor it closely, then." I touch her gently around the catheterization site, and her leg feels soft and compliant. I flick my eyes up to the monitor, where her vital signs are all stable. "I'll be back in here in twenty minutes or so, OK?" I step back out, to check Ms. Brennan's immediate post-op labs, as well as the lab values of a few other patients I'm watching closely.

Twenty minutes later, the discoloration is a little bit worse, a deeper purple, the margins spreading and more turgid. I peel up the dressing, see no blood coming from the actual puncture site, which means that most of the bleeding is internal, leaking from the artery into the soft tissue of the leg. This is ominous, because there's a *lot* of room in an adult human leg, a lot of space for blood to hide before becoming evident. The surgeons had obtained hemostasis, or an effective blood clot at the catheterization site, prior to coming out of the OR, but now, for whatever reason, that access site at the artery has at least partially opened up again. In a calm, pleasant voice, so as not to make Ms. Brennan nervous, I ask Angel to draw another round of labs, and page someone from the Cardiothoracic Surgery team to come by. Then, taking a fresh wad of sterile gauze, I fold the stack into quarters and apply pressure, a *lot* of pressure, to Ms. Brennan's groin over the access site. She winces.

"I'm so sorry, I should have given you some warning, but I'm just going to hold some pressure on your leg here, OK? There's a little bit of bleeding from where the surgeons accessed, but we'll just hold some pressure here until it stops." So many euphemisms we use in medicine. "You're going to feel a little pinch" means, *I'm going to stick this gigantic needle into you now.* "This is going to be a little uncomfortable" means, *This is going to hurt like a motherfucker.* "There's a little bit of bleeding" means, *Don't freak out, but I think you might be bleeding to death.* I give her another little smile, and she smiles back. "I'm being such a bother!" she titters. Is she for real, or something out of Central Casting? I half expect her to reach under her pillow and pull out a pan of oatmeal cookies.

After about fifteen minutes, someone from the Cardiothoracic team shows up—not one of the residents, but Paul, a physician's assistant hired to work overnight. He is blond, clean cut, and fresh scrubbed, one of those annoying people who look completely groomed and put-together at three thirty in the morning. I explain the situation to him, and he offers to take over for me, holding pressure. We do a hand-off like Indiana Jones, replacing the golden idol with a sandbag so as not to let up pressure for a moment, and then Paul, strong and somehow enthusiastic even at this early hour, applies even *more* pressure, in an effort to stem the arterial bleeding and allow a clot to form. Ms. Brennan winces again, and then apologizes. *She* apologizes to *us* for hurting her. Unbelievable. I want to put her in my pocket and take her home.

Now that Paul is here to hold pressure, I can go check the patient in Room 9, whose nurse Ariella I had noticed over the past twenty minutes repeatedly popping her head in and out of Ms. Brennan's room to check whether or not I was free. The patient in Room 9 is Jessica Gomez, a thirty-two-year-old woman who has the dubious honor of being the youngest patient in the CTICU, with a badly regurgitant mitral valve after a failed repair, a valve whose leaflets, instead of closing neatly with every beat of the heart, flail uselessly, allowing too much blood to slosh backward toward the lungs instead of moving forward through the left ventricle and out through the aorta. Right now, Ms. Gomez is not feeling very well. She is breathing with some difficulty, glistening with a light sheen of sweat, and when I listen to her lungs with my stethoscope, they sound wet and bubbly from the bases midway up her chest to the apices. Worrying that fluid is backing up into her lungs, I ask Ariella to give Ms. Gomez a supplemental dose of diuretic immediately, send off an arterial blood gas for analysis, and place her on supplemental oxygen. Taking a quick peek to make sure that there is a Foley catheter in place to measure her urine output, I give Ms. Gomez's foot a squeeze and promise to be back to check on her soon.

Between me and Paul, we have now been holding pressure on Ms. Brennan's cath site for almost an hour, and as we gingerly ease up, things look OK. The leg feels softer, the bruise hasn't increased in size anymore, and her latest blood count from the lab, while a little lower than a few hours ago, is nowhere near the level requiring transfusion. I instruct Ms. Brennan to try and get some rest if she can, keeping her left leg out straight, and ask her if she has any pain. "Oh no dear, just a little sore, but I'm fine, thank you so much." Happy that we seem to have put out this particular fire, I give Angel a thumbs-up and he dims the room lights a touch, pulling up the bedsheet, leaving only Ms. Brennan's left leg uncovered up to the groin.

But half an hour later, the lights are back on, and I am back in the room again. "Look," Angel says succinctly, and shows me Ms. Brennan's leg. The purple mottling has spread to the entire upper thigh now, and as I reapply pressure and palpate the tissue, it feels turgid, like a water balloon filled to capacity. I redouble pressure, hope that it is enough—Ms. Brennan's generous physique gives us a lot of soft tissue to compress, and I don't know how much compressive pressure is getting to the actual artery, to slow the bleeding. I then ask Angel to page Cardiothoracic back immediately, to ask for the fellow this time, and to get the blood up here that has been set aside in the blood bank for Ms. Brennan's surgery. "Tell them to send up two units of packed reds, and order four more," I say, knowing that while the staff at the blood bank is going to give me grief about placing the order for additional blood by phone as opposed to in the computer, I am unable to let up pressure from my bleeding patient and there is nothing else I can do at the moment. Until Angel, Paul, or one of the cardiothoracic surgeons comes back in the room, I am stuck.

It is at this moment that Ariella runs into the room and tells me that Ms. Gomez in Room 9 is now coughing up a copious amount of pink, frothy foam. *Oh Jesus.* She's going into flash pulmonary edema, I'm holding Ms. Brennan's femoral artery to keep her from bleeding to death, and at this moment, I'm the only doctor in the CTICU. "Call Natasha!" I instruct Ariella, naming the ICU fellow on call overnight, who I saw earlier in the evening but who as of an hour ago was helping to troubleshoot a crashing patient with one of the interns in the ICU. "Tell her

I need more hands up here now! And give another dose of Lasix and a dose of Bumex! Turn up the oxygen. What are her PA pressures? Get someone to step in here to hold this leg, I'm coming over there." I crane my head, trying to look out the glass doors of Ms. Brennan's door over to Room 9, where Ms. Gomez is, but it is across the hall and down the hall, and all I can see is the light and the barest sliver of the sink by the door.

Angel rushes back in, I show him where to hold pressure, where to hold it *hard*, indenting the crease of Ms. Brennan's upper thigh a good 2 1/2 inches into her flesh, and run over to Room 9, where, sure enough, Jessica Gomez is coughing bubbly, pinkish exudates into one of the white hospital-issue towels. Ariella reenters with the meds as I read the monitor and listen to Ms. Gomez's lungs (the wet, bubbling sounds are now farther up, past her shoulder blades) and think aloud that we might need to bring the patient's systemic blood pressure down to encourage her blood to flow forward, into her body, rather than backward, into her lungs.

At this, Natasha comes in, still wearing a mask and hat from the line placement she had been supervising with the intern. "What's up?" she asks pleasantly, and I appreciate, though not for the first time, that one feature of a good anesthesiologist is the ability to always stay calm. As briefly as I can, I appraise her of the situation in this room, then tell her what has been happening over in Room 1 with Ms. Brennan, with the newest development indicating a rebleed.

"OK. Good. Let's divide and conquer. I'll handle this patient, you make sure the blood is coming up from Room One and coordinate what to do with the surgeons." The cardiothoracic fellow, another nurse has told me, is on his way.

"Maybe we would do well to page Vascular too," I remark, walking quickly out of the room back toward Ms. Brennan's. If the femoral artery really can't stop leaking, it may be something that requires a trip down to the operating room for exploration and a few stitches into the wall of the artery itself.

"Good thinking, let's get them involved," Natasha says, and I am back across the hall, where Ms. Brennan is lying with her one huge purple leg and apologizing for causing such a *fuss* all night.

The sunrise over the Hudson River is gorgeous under any circumstances, but never more so than at the end of a long night on call, when the breaking daylight seems to say, *You're almost there! The night is almost over! In another hour, the day team will be back, and finally, there will be more people around to take care of all these sick people!* By 6:30 a.m., Ms. Gomez has stabilized, the extra doses of diuretic and extra oxygen having averted disaster at least for the immediate future, and the surgeons are now standing outside her room on morning rounds, coffee in hand, discussing bringing her back to the OR later in the day for a second, and hopefully definitive, mitral valve replacement. At the same time, Ms. Brennan is being wheeled back to the OR herself, a bag of red blood cells hanging over her head. The stretcher is being pushed by two nurses, one of the Vascular residents, and an Anesthesia resident at the head of the bed, who warns those steering the feet, "Watch out! Watch out!" before the bed clips the wheeled chart rack in the hallway with a crash. Ms. Brennan, looking a little pale but otherwise doing well, apologizes, of course.

"Well that was an exciting night," Natasha deadpans, sidling up to me as I watch the team wheel down the hall.

"Yeah, a little *too* exciting for me," I respond. "There was a moment there where...when I was the only one here...Anyway, I'm glad you were able to come up so quickly. Thank god you were here."

"No," she says emphatically, "thank god *you* were here." And around us, the day team starts arriving, loud and chatty, smelling of shampoo and shaving cream, full of coffee and energy and ready to start their morning.

Opposing Interests

One morning, still in the Cardiothoracic ICU, I happen upon one of the surgical fellows checking his e-mail. He is opening up some picture files that he has been sent, a series of photos of a baby in a pastel pink sleeper who looks to be about three or four months old. I ask him if they are pictures of his daughter.

"Yeah, that's her." He beams proudly. "I work so much that my wife e-mails me these pictures. That way, I get to see her once in a while."

Depressing.

The key difficulty in balancing work and real life

is that the needs of one are often diametrically opposed to the needs of the other. In medicine one thinks more often about the demands of work interfering with the needs of tending to home and family—the demanding hours away from home, the stress, the fatigue, the rigors of the day that lead the mind back to the wards, even when at home. We try to compartmentalize in so much as it is possible, trying to keep the two worlds apart, but given how all-consuming each can be, this separation can be difficult to achieve. And occasionally, it's not just the demands of work that interfere with life at home. Sometimes, it can even be the other way around.

* * *

David Barbaro is blasting off.

Of course, this is a euphemism. "Blasting off" is just another way of saying that David is dying. He's a child with relapsed acute lymphocytic leukemia (ALL) who, over the course of the past two years, has failed several courses of chemotherapy and radiation and most recently has undergone an ultimately unsuccessful bone marrow transplant. He has reached the end of the road when it comes to curative measures, and now the Oncology team's efforts are centered around palliation, or relief of suffering. And this is where I get involved. It is the beginning of my third year of Anesthesia residency, and I am spending the week rotating with the Pediatric Pain service.

I learn more about David's story on rounds. After coming to the difficult conclusion that David's cancer is in its terminal stage, the Oncology team had many discussions with the family to assess how they wanted to proceed with his medical care. There were those voices in the Greek chorus who felt at this point, overly aggressive measures would have little if any benefit and only prolong the pain of an already protracted battle with the disease. Why extend the child's suffering when the outcome was certain? David's parents felt differently, however. They wanted, as my attending, Dr. Bill Schechter, put it, "the full court press." Certainly, they wanted David to get pain medication, as much as he needed to be comfortable, even to the point of extreme sedation. But if the time came that David stopped breathing, or that his heart stopped beating, they wanted everything possible done to bring him back. Everything, including the violence of a full resuscitation, with chest compressions and an intubation. What they want, in essence, is just a little more time with their son. David is just two years old.

David was getting palliative chemo for the last few weeks—that is to say, chemotherapy where the goal is no longer to cure, but merely reduce the symptoms of the disease. But even that has been stopped in recent days. At first, after the chemo was discontinued, the cancer cells lay low, quiescent for the time being. But then, like cockroaches peeking out from cracks in the wall, they started appearing in his peripheral blood work. Just a few darting by at first, then more, then exponentially more. Over the past few days, his white blood count has skyrocketed from the relatively normal value of about 10 to the elevated 31, to the higher yet 44, to now the astronomical value of 91. Almost all of these white blood cells are the immature cells known in shorthand as blasts, which are the hallmark of ALL. Hence, in oncologic parlance, David is "blasting off." At this point, his life expectancy can be counted not in months or weeks, but in days.

We walk into David's room this morning and, as usual, the room is dim, shades drawn. His mother, weary and rumpled, sees us and smiles in greeting. David himself does not react, except to lie there, drumming his fist on his forehead, a strangely adult-looking gesture to see in a toddler. His head hurts. It has been hurting him for the past week. It is unclear what exactly underlies this pain—scans to date show no definitive intracranial mass that anyone can pinpoint, and other causes have similarly been excluded. The one theory that anyone can come up with at this point is that it is the bones of the skull itself that are causing his pain. Like the bones of the femur and the pelvis, the skull too contains marrow, which in David has gone haywire and is churning out millions and millions of deranged immature blood cells, machinery gone amok. The pressure of the marrow, packed with these immature cells, could be exerting pressure on the bone, causing David to repeatedly complain of a headache. That is one thought. Or, we could just chalk it up as one more of the many, many things that we don't understand and can't explain.

This morning, David has visitors. One of his mother's oldest friends is visiting, and she brings along her two children, a six-year-old son and her four-year-old daughter. Unlike the rest of us, who instinctively soften our voices, walk more slowly, fold our hands together as we walk into David's room (which has, to be honest, with its dim lighting and religious pamphlets and tracts posted on every wall, the feel of a mausoleum), the visiting children are rambunctious. They do not seem afraid, as I would think they might, of the pumps, the miles of tubing, of David's appearance. As I watch, the boy crawls into David's bed, literally on top of him, and wraps his arms around the toddler, giving him a kiss on the cheek.

Dr. Schechter is now talking to David's mother in a low voice, asking her about David's night, how well the modifications to his pain regimen have been working. But I can't quite hear all of what is being said, because the two children are scampering around the room and shrieking exuberantly about a basketball set that they have brought along to play with—a large hoop rimmed by netting and a stash of brightly colored foam balls. David, who I have never seen open his eyes in the several times that I have been by his room, is watching these proceedings with some interest.

His mother's friend comes over, sits on his bed. "Who wants to play basketball?" she asks cheerfully. "Me," David says in his small, rough voice. She hands him one of the balls, a purple one, and he makes a game effort to loft it into the netting.

Dr. Schechter wraps it up with David's mother, the two of them having made some joint decisions to increase the levels of David's pain medication, and to further discuss his headaches with the Oncology service. Then, excusing ourselves, we walk out of the room and close the door gently. "Did you see that?" my attending asks softly. "The kid is dying and still he wants to play."

I open my mouth to say something intelligent and clinical—maybe to make some remark about "the resilience of children," or one of those stock phrases you always hear—and surprise myself by suddenly dissolving into tears. Embarrassed, I grab a paper towel and start furtively swiping at my eyes.

Dr. Schechter walks over to the nursing station, where, saying nothing, he sits down and starts filling out some paperwork. Grateful for the silence and not particularly wanting to make excuses for myself, I sit down too and try to think about something else. We sit there quietly for what feels like a long time, with the sound of medication pumps beeping, telephones ringing, and hushed voices of the rounding infectious disease team down the hallway create a pleasant background distraction. I check some lab values on the computer to get my mind back to work, but against my will think suddenly of Cal holding out a ball to me, demanding, "Mama, throw it!" And there, I'm crying again.

One of the nurses notices. "Are you OK?" she asks, concerned. Again, I start to try and speak, embarrassed, wanting to apologize and cover up, tell her that *I'm OK, totally fine, I just don't know what's wrong with me today.* But before I can say anything, Dr. Schechter breaks in instead and tells her firmly, "No. I don't think any of us are OK."

Then, pressing his lips together tightly, he continues writing his note, which outlines the escalation of David's anesthetic infusion, which will hopefully keep him awake and in as little pain as possible until he dies.

Earlier, he told me about David specifically and also about palliative care in general: "What we don't often talk to parents about is the fact that we can actually help *choose* how their child will die." He was discussing children with end-stage cancer. "For instance, a child like this could die after having a seizure. A child like this could have his platelets drop and drop and suddenly just bleed out from everywhere." He paused, perhaps remembering one such end. "Dying of respiratory depression from opioids is a gentle death. Dying of a massive hemorrhage is a violent one. We can't change the fact that these kids are going to die, but we can sometimes control the way that these deaths will take place."

He paused, looked at me. "Those images, those moments, are going to be with the parents forever. *Forever.* They will *always* remember this. We want to be able to give them the option to avoid that kind of...ugliness. We can't always, but we can try." I thought about the kinds of bad death that Dr. Schechter was talking about. And it occured to me that at the very end, perhaps it is the parents and the caretakers who ultimately need the palliation even more than the patients themselves.

He finished by saying in his quiet way, "Perhaps the best thing for everyone sometimes is just for the patients to be comfortable and pain-free on a morphine drip, and just let the parents crawl into bed and hold them until they fall asleep."

When Dr. Schechter walked away to check a note in the chart, my coresident turned to me and asked, "But at what point does that cross over from *accepting* the effects of the pain medications to actually *causing* the death?" She frowned. "It's sort of an invisible line."

"I don't really know." I thought about this some more. "And honestly, I hope I never really have to know except in a purely academic sense." And while I know that it is my job to learn these things, part of me wanted nothing more than to run away from all this, bury myself back in the comfort of hard science and pharmacology and theory, and try to forget that any of this could ever happen to *any* family, let alone a family so similar to mine.

* * *

I had the chance to leave work early, and back at home, I am enjoying a rare early afternoon with Cal. Now two years old, he has started attending a biweekly playgroup, which we conceived of as his separation training wheels. He will be starting preschool full-time the following fall.

As much as I would have loved to take Cal to his first day of "school," this had to be another one of the milestones I hear about secondhand. With my work schedule, there's no way I even entertained the idea of being the one to bring him in to class that first day. So we did the best we could. Joe, now an attending with more flexible hours, arranged his work schedule so that he would be able to take Cal in himself. I talked to Cal about school, read to him endlessly from *Curious George's First Day of School*, and laid out his photo op–worthy clothes the night before. Cal has now been attending class for about a month, and has long since stopped crying after being dropped off by our nanny. I am told that when he walks in the door, he immediately runs over to the teacher, to whom he has become attached, and starts playing with the toy trains and puzzles in the room in the short period of time before the organized activities begin. I love hearing these stories, try to picture the classroom from these descriptions, having never actually seen the facilities myself.

After work each day, eager and hungry for the details of his day, I interrogate Cal.

ME : Did you go to class today? Did you have fun?

HE : The kitties are happy. They go to sleep when it's dark outside.

ME : I...yes. You read a story about kitties in class?

HE : *(As though speaking to someone who is not very bright)* No.

ME : Oh. Well...did you listen to the teachers? And play with the other children? What did you have for snack?

HE : Daddy go to working now.

ME : Yes, Daddy's at work. But how was school, *school*? Did you have fun?

HE : I'm going to ride the bicycle so fast. *(Runs off to ride his bicycle so fast)*

Two years ago, when Cal was little more than a newborn and I was just a week back at work after my maternity leave, I had a conversation with Furious George, one of my senior residents, a gruff redhead who also happened to be the father of two young children, though he has since expanded his brood to three. Looking for something to assuage the guilt I was feeling, I asked him whether or not it got easier, the process of leaving your child home for such long hours each day while you worked. "He's still so *little*," I fretted, the late hour at work and the stress of reentry leading to this rare unsolicited outpouring. "I feel like I'm missing out on *everything*." I paused and waited for him to convince me that this was not the case.

He did not. Instead, he fixed me with a deep glare and told me, "Don't fool yourself into thinking you're not missing anything. You're missing *plenty*. You're not there most of the day, and you're asleep most of the time that you're home. I wasn't there when my kids learned to roll over or when my son took his first steps." And then he shrugged. "But they'll do all those things again and again, and you can be there then."

I think about this now, more than two years later, as I am trying to get the story of Cal's day at school from this uncooperative historian. I want to hear everything, every last detail of what the classroom looks like, how it's lit, whether or not it smells like poster paints and crumbly construction paper like I remember from my own nursery school classroom. I want to hear about the other children, what their names are, what they look like, whether or not they are polite and gentle, or whether or not Gus the Overlarge Two-Year-Old plays too rough. In other words, *I want to be there*, if not in person, then at least in my mind's eye, to be able to be at work taking care of patients and be with my son at the same time.

But since I cannot, all I can do, the best I *can* do, is to be here right now, home this evening after work. I can be here, scrubs and stethoscope shed, hospital smell showered off, and laugh as my two-and-a-half-year-old son pedals in circles around me, yelling exuberantly, "Hey Mommy! Hey Mommy! Hey Mommy!" over and over again, so loud that it makes my ears hurt.

7 . CODES

I'M IN FRONT OF THE VENDING MACHINE on the third floor, fingering my dollar bill and weighing the choice between Pop-Tarts and a bag of chips somewhat alarmingly labeled "Doritos eXtreme!" when I get the page. ARREST STAT, 8 HUDSON SOUTH, screams the text message on the screen, as simultaneously, the same message starts blaring from the hospital-wide speaker system overhead. Feeling a little like Batman spotting a bat-silhouetted searchlight in the sky, I pocket my money and start running. A gaggle of surgical residents standing nearby, taking in my sprint and the large fluorescent orange arrest bag on my shoulder, exchange glances. "That had better not be one of my patients trying to die," one remarks casually.

Elevators in this hospital being somewhat less than reliable, I opt instead to run up the stairs, gear in tow. From the third floor to the fifth floor, I lope up the steps, filled with purpose, taking two at a time, keys and pagers jangling, threatening with each bounce to take my pants down with them. From the fifth through the seventh floor, I start to take the steps one at a time, but still briskly, in emergency mode. By the time I get up to the eighth floor, I am using the banister to pull myself up, face purple, quadriceps burning, the huge arrest bag heavier than ever. Speaking of cardiac arrests, I feel like I'm about to have one myself.

After taking a moment to orient myself coming out of the stairwell, I start running for the nursing station from where the code was called. The ward clerk, seeing my telltale orange bag, silently points me down the hall. I don't have to ask her which room—clearly it's the one with all the people milling outside. Pushing my way in, I see a bed, a patient's feet bouncing on it with the force of the CPR he is receiving, surrounded by a forest of residents and nurses. "Anesthesia!" I try to shout, my face still plummy, voice thin and reedy from my sprint.

No one turns around. "Another round of epi," the senior resident indicates to his intern, as another resident struggles to get central venous access at the patient's groin. I am closer now, and I see that the patient is an elderly man, obese, his skin as gray as poured cement. He is unresponsive to these ministrations, does not fight as one of the nurses attempts to ventilate him with a bag valve mask.

I take a deeper breath and try to force my voice into a lower, more carrying register. "ANESTHESIA!"

The crowd turns, and starts parting. *Anesthesia.*

Anesthesia's here. Give her some room. I weave in through the crowd and make my way to the head of the bed. I look to the resident standing by the foot of the bed, the one who has been shouting orders and looks most in charge, and start to unzip the arrest bag as I ask him, "So what's the story here?"

He starts scanning the crowd. As the senior arrest resident, he does not know much of this patient's history. "Does anyone know this patient?" he addresses the throng. Everybody looks around. The resident doing chest compressions, looking winded, motions to another resident across the bed from her to take over, and they trade off.

Finally, an intern speaks up. "I don't know him too well, he just came up from the ER." And with that caveat in place, she launches into her bullet-point history. "Seventy-nine-year-old man, prior history of MI and stroke, came to the ER complaining of dizziness—I think—admitted for observation, found unresponsive about ten minutes ago." She adds again, apologetically, "I really don't know him that well, he just got up here."

"Can we reassess for a pulse, please?" the senior resident asks, and the chest compressions stop as three people separately reach to palpate for a pulse on either side of the man's groin, and over the right carotid artery in his neck. "No pulse," someone finally says after a few seconds. "Resume compressions," the senior resident says, and the team falls on the man again.

I am taking out my equipment—an endotracheal tube, my laryngoscope—and I turn around to make sure that I have suction set up. I have medications that I usually use to induce at least some level of anesthesia in patients prior to intubation, but from the look of this guy, he doesn't really need any anesthetic. In fact, if he were any *more* unresponsive, he would be dead. Actually, technically, he *is* dead. I flip open my laryngoscope, slip it down the patient's throat, and look in.

The patient's mouth is cold and stiff, unlike those of my patients in the OR. It occurs to me that though we have so much equipment to determine whether patients are alive or dead, really all you have to do is touch them. This patient's tissues are cool and clammy with the consistency of refrigerated clay. I lift my scope and look in. There are his vocal cords, bouncing in and out of view with the force of the chest compressions. After chasing them around with my tube for a few seconds, I look up and ask the resident, "Sorry, could you stop chest compressions for just...one second?" He obliges, and, moving target stilled, I am able to pass the tube with a minimum of fuss. I hook the tube up to my bag, ventilate, and see the chest rise. Someone is already listening to both sides of the chest with a stethoscope. "It's good," she says, meaning the air movement sounds equal on both sides, and that the tube is in the right place. *Swish.* Three points.

"Does anyone here object to us calling it?" the senior resident suddenly says, his voice rising above the rest. Three people are feeling for a pulse again, finding nothing. There is a brief silence. "OK then, thanks everyone," the senior says breezily, the voice of a tennis player thanking his opponent for a good game. "Time of death, 22:53." Everyone nods in agreement, equipment is removed, and the senior members of the team start filing out while the juniors commence cleaning up the mess that has accumulated. "Someone needs to call the family," I hear one person say as they exit. "What's this guy's name again?" says another, presumably looking for the patient's chart. I pack up my own gear, thank everyone for their help, and walk out of the room myself. The patient continues lying there, being dead, my endotracheal tube doing nothing to make him less so.

As a senior Anesthesia resident, in my third and final year of training, I am now often responsible for holding what is known as the "code pager," which is one of a series of alerts that goes off anytime anyone at the hospital requires emergent resuscitation in the event of cardiac arrest, respiratory arrest, or trauma. As the anesthesiologist on the scene, my main job is to manage the airway, assessing the need for intubation and securing the patient's ability to ventilate their lungs by whatever means possible.

The majority of adult "codes" (as we call the arrests) are pretty similar. Usually by the time Anesthesia is called, the patient is basically dead, a fact that cannot be changed by any amount of resuscitation; or they are *almost* dead, in a twilight limbo that can be prolonged by any number of industrial-strength drugs and a ventilator. There are times when patients recover from such events—these are obviously the success stories that we all relish—but much of the time, the remainder of the patient's story is a slow-motion version of the same code, only played out over days or weeks. In other words, we save the patients from a merciful quick death so that they can die a horrific slow one.

As the anesthesiologist called to do the stat intubation, I really only see a very small part of the patient's story. We as the anesthesiologists don't know the patients before we tube them, we've never met their families, we don't continue to follow them after the tube is in, and for the most part, we never really find out what happens to them in the long run. All we have with them is those few minutes, that window of chaos, the fulcrum between death and the alternative. Oftentimes, knowing less about the story and having fewer emotional ties to the patient makes things easier.

But sometimes it does not.

* * *

I run into the room where I have been called, on the oncology ward up on the fifth floor. The patient is a man, and it is difficult to tell how old he is, because there's very little of him left. He is utterly emaciated, every bone, joint, and sinew showing clearly through his papery skin, and with each labored breath, I can see the muscles between the ribs straining. He could be fifty-five, he could be ninety-five, it is difficult to say.

"Anesthesia?" I ask, not even knowing whom I am addressing. There is no one in the room but this patient, his sleeping roommate, and a middle-aged woman in a bright pink jogging suit, who stands there facing the patient, back to the door. JUICY, reads a string of rhinestones linked across her ample rear. *Doesn't that hurt her when she sits down?* I wonder. But instead, I say, "Is there...I mean, did someone call for a stat intubation?"

At this moment, a resident breezes in from the hallway, the patient's chart in hand. "Oh good, you're here," he says, recognizing my neon orange luggage. "We called you for this gentleman. End-stage colon cancer, increasing respiratory distress. But just hold on a second. We're not really sure if we want you to do anything yet."

"You're not sure if..." I look at the man, who looks as ready to stop breathing as anyone I've ever seen. "What's the problem exactly?"

After a glance at the bedazzled-jogging-suit woman, who I have inferred is the patient's daughter, the resident tersely recaps. The patient has end-stage colon cancer and is receiving palliative care to make his inevitable passing as comfortable as possible. He is demented, and all medical decisions are being made by his son, who is currently in Baltimore. However, his other three children all agree that in his situation, their father should not be subjected to the organized violence of an aggressive resuscitation, that it is not what their father would have wanted, and they have been negotiating with the holdout sibling in hopes of making their father DNR. They were still in the middle of these talks when their father took a turn for the worse and it became clear that the choice was either to intubate him and have him die soon on a venti-

lator, or *not* intubate him and have him die sooner
without one. And here we are.

"There's no DNR in the chart," the resident says
now, flipping through the sheets of paper in the back
of the patient's substantial chart. "We are legally obligated to resuscitate him if there's no DNR order
from his medical proxy." The patient's daughter is on
her cell phone already, dialing a series of numbers
in rapid succession with fingernails that look like
fuchsia-lacquered Fritos. She lifts the phone to her
ear and waits impatiently.

"Duane," she shouts into the phone when someone finally picks up, pronouncing the name with two
syllables, "it's me. He's looking really bad now, and
they're saying that they're going to put the tube
down his throat now unless you sign the papers. So
what now?" She pauses, listens. "They said they're
going to stick a *tube* in him and put him on a *breathing* machine. They might need to give him *shocks*
and do CPR on him and beat on his *chest*. We don't
want that. Lateesha and Kendra and me, we don't
want that. Tell them that they don't have to do it."
Another pause. "He wouldn't *want* it, Duane! Why
you tellin' them...just *talk* to them! There's a doctor right here! Here!" And with that, she thrusts the
cell phone into the hands of the unsuspecting resident, who is so surprised that he almost fumbles the
pass-off.

"Mister"—the resident takes a peek at the name
on the patient's chart—"Brown? We haven't met, I'm
Dr. Singh, one of the residents taking care of your father." And again, he details the situation, not skimp-

ing words. "If we intubate your father, in all likelihood, he will never come off the breathing machine.
If he arrests—that is, if his heart stops beating—we
will have to give him some very strong medications,
and we may have to shock his heart with electric-
ity. We may need to do CPR, which involves forceful
compressions to the front of the chest. In a man
your father's age, it is not uncommon that we might
break some ribs in the process, and that could be very
painful for him." He is being candid, blunt, in a way
that we rarely are in medicine.

I understand what he's doing. The resident wants
Duane Brown to make the decision he has been entrusted to make as his father's medical proxy, but
he also wants Duane Brown to make what he as the
doctor feels is the *right* decision. I have seen this
strategy countless times in countless different incar-
nations. It even comes into play when presenting the
different options available to patients for anesthesia. An attending once illustrated this for me using a
choice between general anesthesia and a spinal anesthetic as an example. "You could either have a simple
spinal anesthetic," he said, speaking to me playing
the role of the patient, "in which we numb you completely from the ribs down and give you some sedation [*beatific expression*], allowing you to be sleepy
and pain-free during the surgery with fewer post-
operative complications [*big smile, nodding, thumbs-
up*] and avoiding the need to do general anesthesia
[*frown*]. With general anesthesia [*frown again*] we
would have to stick a TUBE down your THROAT and
give you GAS to breathe, which will make you nau-

seous and groggy afterward, and might delay your discharge from the recovery room." He then made this alternative presentation: "We could either give you a spinal anesthetic, in which we stick a long, sharp NEEDLE into your BACK [*stabbing motion not dissimilar to prison shanking*] near your SPINAL CORD to inject local anesthesia around the nerves, which comes with potential complications such as bleeding, blood pressure instability, and PERMANENT NERVE DAMAGE, and which in the end might not even work one hundred percent for the surgery. Or, [*clasping hands, sighing happily*] we could just give you general anesthesia and have you drift off totally to sleep, waking you up at the end when it's all finished. So, it's your decision. What do you think?"

Maybe it's that Duane Brown is on the phone with the resident, and thus spared the most graphic of the possible pantomime that could be employed in explaining the current situation. Or maybe he just has stronger convictions than the average health care proxy on what the desires of his father would be in this situation, even in the face of this multipronged attack from the doctors and his own siblings. Most likely, however—and I have seen this before too—he just doesn't want to be the one making the decision. If his father is dying of cancer, he can come to accept that. But if his father died here, tonight, because he, Duane, has told us to withhold our aggressive life support—*that*, he could not cope with.

The resident hangs up the phone a short time later. He is struggling to maintain a neutral tone of voice, but his disgust with the decision is clear. He looks up to where I am standing, near the head of the patient's bed. "You might as well go ahead and tube him."

"Yeah? Are you sure?"

"It's what the son wants."

I set up, and within two minutes, the tube is in. It is an easy intubation, almost grotesquely so given the difficulty of the decision that preceded it. I don't dare to give him more than that barest whiff of sedating medication, so tremulous is this patient's grasp on life at this point, and he does not flinch as I slide the cold metal of the laryngoscope down his parched mouth, or as I pass the plastic tubing past the vocal cords into his trachea. I breathe for him, see his chest rise, the condensation on the plastic—the tube is in. The respiratory therapist has appeared, seemingly out of nowhere, and is setting up the ventilator. The patient's daughter, distraught at this latest turn, sobs in the hallway. The patient, looking more skeletal than ever, heaves, trembles, and, breathing shallowly, accepts the tube.

I feel like an accomplice to a crime.

* * *

It is mid-November, close to Thanksgiving, when I am called to a stat intubation in the Medical ICU. I round the corner and find myself in the middle of what appears to be a very large crowd. The patient I have been called to intubate has anywhere between fifteen to twenty family members present, and all of them appear to be crying.

Stepping between the bodies and trying to weave my way into the room, I spy the familiar face of one of my medical school classmates, Natalie, who I know has recently finished her Internal Medicine residency and is now working in the ICU as one of the pulmonology fellows. She sees me and helps me into the room.

"Hey," I say, still out of breath from my sprint to the MICU. "What's all this?" I gesture globally, including the patient, the crowd, and the respiratory machinery in one grand arc of my arm.

Natalie looks down at the patient, who appears to be a woman in her late sixties, a penumbra of silvery hair fanning out over the pillow, and explains. Mrs. Santana is a woman with idiopathic pulmonary fibrosis, a condition in which the tissue of the lungs becomes thickened and stiff over time, impairing the ability to oxygenate the blood and thus the body. She was admitted several days ago for increasing difficulty breathing, and has been on escalating degrees of respiratory support over the course of this hospitalization, moving from first supplemental oxygen, to CPAP, to BiPAP, in which pressure is blown into the lungs with each breath, only one step away from actually being intubated and on a ventilator. Despite these measures, her blood gas measurements have been deteriorating, and it is becoming apparent that she will need to be intubated sometime soon, within the next hour. It has been explained to the family, Natalie continues, as Mrs. Santana listens and nods, that barring a lung transplant, her changes of coming off the ventilator are slim.

I introduce myself as "Dr. Au from the Anesthesia team," and tell Mrs. Santana that I'm going to be putting a breathing tube in her mouth to help her lungs breathe. I reassure her that I will make sure she is asleep and comfortable, and that she won't feel a thing. Again, she nods, her lips moving behind the clear plastic of the oversized BiPAP mask.

Looking up at her oxygen saturation and seeing that the numbers are holding for now, I look out again into the hallway, where I see three generations of family members watching, their faces almost pushed up against the glass. Knowing that in all likelihood Mrs. Santana will be receiving sedation after intubation and will no longer be able to speak with the endotracheal tube through her vocal cords, I ask Natalie if the family would like a few minutes before I proceed. She agrees, and I step out into the hallway, allowing Mrs. Santana to exchange a few words with them before I take away her voice.

After about twelve minutes, the last of the family exits, eyes red, damp tissues clutched to the palms of their hands. I reenter the room and draw the curtains. Setting up, I ready my equipment and take off the BiPAP mask, which releases with a gust of air. "Mrs. Santana, I'm going to help you go to sleep now. When you wake up, you're going to have a tube in your mouth." She smiles, her face still pink with the imprint of that mask, and pats my arm, her hands soft and warm. "Thank you, my darling," she whispers, her voice hoarse.

With a push of my induction agent, her eyes start to flutter, and she slowly becomes unconscious, stops breathing. I open Mrs. Santana's mouth, look inside, and carefully slip in my tube. We ventilate. The tube is in.

"So, how's the baby doing?" I ask Natalie, as I tape the tube into place. Natalie has just recently returned from maternity leave, having had a baby girl three months prior.

"She's great, getting big. How's yours?"

"Oh, man, not so much of a baby anymore. Last week, he started shaving," I joke. We exchange small talk about our children for a few minutes as I squeeze the bag—breathing for Mrs. Santana by hand as the ventilator is being set up—asking after each other's family and catching up on mutual med school acquaintances. Then, duty dispensed, I pack up my equipment and exit the ICU, as Natalie heads on back to the family waiting room to inform the Santanas that their matriarch has been successfully placed on a ventilator, which will hopefully buy her some time for the slim chance that a set of lungs becomes available for transplant.

As I walk back toward the operating rooms, replaying this last scene in my head, it occurs to me that somehow by repetitive exposure and some sort of gradual weathering of the psyche, what once may have seemed to be life defining and critical for us in medical school has now become mundane, commonplace. I'm not sure if this protective mechanism is a good thing or a bad thing.

* * *

It is 9:32 at night, and I am trying to convince the members of my call team to eat their dinner out of emesis basins.

The emesis basins are made of pink plastic, molded into a curved colon shape (the punctuation type of colon, not the feces-compacting type of colon) meant to be used by patients who, for a variety of reasons, need a receptacle into which to vomit. The problem is this: we have ordered Mexican food for dinner. A *lot* of Mexican food. The delivery guys have forgotten to bring us plates. There are no paper plates anywhere that we can find. My team seems to have no issue with eating dinner prepared in a questionably clean back kitchen, yet when it comes to eating rice and beans out of a patient vomit basin, for some reason everyone's an inspector for the Board of Health.

"They're *clean* emesis basins!" I take an illustrative forkful of food from my own pink plastic receptacle, which, it should be noted, is exactly the right size for a personal portion of grilled chicken fajita with a side of rice. "They're *disposable*! It's not like I'm suggesting that you eat out of one that some guy actually *puked* in or anything." I'm clearly improving everyone's appetite with my pep talk.

Eventually, I convince about half of my team to eat from the pink receptacles, leaving the other half to dine off the clear plastic lids of the food containers. "I would keep those basins handy though, even after you're finished," I tell my team in a low voice. "Someone on call last week got food poisoning from the takeout at this place. I'm just saying."

It is my third and final year of Anesthesia residency, and on this night, I am the team captain. As TC, I am in charge of overseeing the residents of the call team, all activity in the ORs, as well as managing the patients in the Post Anesthesia Care Unit (or PACU), which, overnight, can hold up to a dozen patients. In addition, of course, I am holding the arrest pager and must be ready at any moment to drop what I am doing should any patient in the hospital require intubation overnight.

Whenever I am on TC call, I make sure I am wearing my sneakers, because I do a lot of running.

I am making my rounds though the PACU when I see one of the Vascular Surgery residents unlocking one of the patients' stretchers and starting to push him down the hall. Since residents usually don't transport patients unless there is something precarious or critical about their clinical situation, I catch up to him and ask him what's going on.

The resident, a pleasant and (need it be said) overworked junior named Dan, responds that the patient is being taken to CT scan for evaluation of a developing retroperitoneal hematoma, a growing blood collection behind the organs in his pelvis. The patient had a device placed in order to stent open his femoral artery earlier that day, and there is reason to believe that he is having some bleeding as a result of that surgery, bleeding all the more difficult to assess because it is all collecting internally, where it is impossible to monitor with the naked eye. His blood counts are dropping, however, and his heart rate is going up in an effort to compensate, so they are taking him to CT scan to evaluate the extent of the bleed. The patient, a neatly groomed older man named Benjamin Lozada, lies on his stretcher, smiling mildly and nodding along, as though to confirm that yes, Dan has gotten the story right.

Dan returns without fanfare about half an hour later, pushing the still beatific Mr. Lozada. "So, what did the scan show?" I ask, catching up to the two of them.

"Significant left retroperitoneal hematoma," he reports back, parking the stretcher back into position and giving the brake lever a hard *thump* to lock it into place.

"Whoa, what does that mean, 'significant'?" I ask, "How 'significant' is 'significant'? Did they give you a volume?"

"I think they said seven by ten centimeters, something like that," Dan reports while checking his pager, which seems to be squawking alarmingly at increasingly frequent intervals.

Holding my fingers apart to estimate a clot seven by ten centimeters in size, I reply, "That sounds pretty big, Dan. What's the plan here, then? Are you guys taking him back into surgery?"

"No," Dan says, reaching for the phone on the wall and dialing a string of numbers rapidly. "My attending just wants to watch him. He says that it'll probably stabilize, and that he'll be fine." Knowing that as a junior resident Dan does not actually have any say in the treatment or management of this patient—his job is more that of a foot soldier, carrying out the orders issued to him from on high—I turn my attention to the patient, who is being hooked back up to his PACU monitors by the nursing team.

"Too much excitement, isn't it, Mr. Lozada?" I joke. He smiles back at me, with a benign facial expression that seems to say, *What can you do?* Looking him over with a more critical eye, I take stock of his situation. Vital signs are stable, though his heart rate seems on the high side at 92 beats per minute, probably to compensate for the decreased blood volume. He has only one IV in place, and a small one at that, insufficient for giving any sort of fluid or blood in a resuscitative capacity, as we might need to. He has terrible vascular disease, with plaques hardening the arteries throughout his entire body, and as a result, has no palpable pulses anywhere. In fact, even with the Doppler, which uses ultrasound to assess for pulsatile blood flow, I can only measure a pulse in one of his four extremities—his left foot. This is the only way that we are able to measure Mr. Lozada's blood pressure, by placing the cuff on his calf, cycling the cuff, and listening with the Doppler for the sound of pulsatile flow to disappear, then reappear.

My inclination at this point is to put in an arterial line, a small catheter that continually evaluates a patient's blood pressure with each beat of his heart; but on the other hand, if we are unable to get in the line and blow the artery, I also will have left us with no good way to determine his blood pressure at all. So after discussing the plan with my attending, I struggle to get in a larger IV (with the extent of his vascular disease, he has no viable veins left, either, which makes things difficult—I finally end up getting access on the inside of his left ankle), give him a good-sized bolus of extra fluid to compensate for the blood loss, and instruct the nurse to record his Dopplered blood pressure at least every fifteen minutes, knowing that a rising heart rate and dropping blood pressure will be one of the first signs that the hidden bleeding has not stopped and that things are going south.

About an hour later, his new round of blood tests come back from the lab. Mr. Lozada's blood counts, while on the lower end as we might expect, are not critically low and, more importantly, have not changed in the past four hours. However, as he is an older man with some history of cardiac disease, and with borderline blood counts and a questionably expanding hematoma, I am inclined to transfuse some blood. So following the accepted medical chain of communication, resident-to-resident, I call Dan. "Dan, how do you feel about transfusing this guy?" I ask, by way of greeting, when he answers my page.

"Well..." He sounds hesitant. "My attending doesn't want him to be transfused until his crit is down to twenty-seven. His last two crits were around thirty." A "crit," short for hematocrit, is the percentage of blood volume occupied by red blood cells, the oxygen-carrying component of the blood. A normal hematocrit is closer to 40, though most patients do fine with crits of mid-30s or, depending on how sick they are, even lower.

"But with a significant retroperitoneal hematoma?

He doesn't want him to get blood?" I know I am putting Dan in a difficult situation—he has been given his orders that he is to carry out—but I am in a difficult situation as well. As the senior resident running the PACU, Mr. Lozada is *my* patient for the night, but my efforts and treatment plans can still be vetoed by the orders of his primary team of surgeons, most of whom, with the exception of Dan, are not physically in the hospital.

To his credit, Dan offers to call his attending surgeon at home, no small feat of bravery, especially given the fact that it is now 2:00 a.m. However, when he calls me back fifteen minutes later, it is only to tell me that the attending surgeon's plan for his patient has not changed. Stay the course. Watchful waiting. He is to receive no blood.

I walk by Mr. Lozada's bed again. He is still awake, looking chipper. His blood pressure is holding, his heart rate slower after the fluid bolus he has been given. His urine output over the past few hours has been good, indicating adequate blood flow to the kidneys. Despite my apprehension, I think to myself that the attending surgeon may be right. This certainly isn't the first time he's seen a complication like this, and he has been in practice decades more than I have. So I let it go, deciding to check Mr. Lozada's blood count again in a few hours with a morning round of lab work.

By the morning, Mr. Lozada is one of only two patients remaining in the PACU, the rest of the herd having found their ways upstairs to rooms and beds sometime throughout the night. He is still holding his own, vital signs rock stable, and waves at me as I pass by. His nurse tells me that a bed in the step-down unit (a sort of staged close-observation unit, one level down from intensive care) has opened up, and that Mr. Lozada will be moving upstairs shortly. With that expansive, euphoric feeling that comes at the end of a long night on call, I smile with relief. It's almost over. Mr. Lozada and I have both sur-vived the night.

I survey my tidy PACU with satisfaction and de-cide that I can step away for Grand Rounds, a teach-ing conference held in an auditorium on the first floor every Thursday morning. All my patients are stable, I am going off-duty in less than an hour, and so I feel fine stepping away to a lecture at which I am easily reachable. But not safe enough to leave without my big orange arrest bag. I carry it with me into the au-ditorium, so as not to jinx myself. I am still holding the code pager, after all.

About forty minutes into the conference, I get a page. Not an emergency arrest page, just a regular page on my personal pager to the PACU. I call back, wondering what it could possibly be at this point in the morning, with only two patients in the PACU and no ORs running.

One of the nurses picks up. "We were moving Lozada to go to his room upstairs, and he became kind of confused and unresponsive. He's sort of starting to wake up a little bit now, though. I think everything is fine." I am somewhat reassured by the latter, but the former sounds alarming. I tell the nurse that I will be back upstairs in three minutes and grab my arrest bag, turning heads in Grand Rounds with my rapid exit and flash of neon orange.

Things are not fine.

By the time I reach the PACU, Mr. Lozada is confused, slurring his speech, breathing laboriously. The nurses have moved him back from the transport stretcher to his bed, and he is slumped over to his right side. I ask him some quick, direct questions and get only unintelligible, groaning responses, then nothing at all. His blood pressure cuff is cycling, cycling, but we are not getting any blood pressure reading. His heart rate is in the 100s. His eyes, which had been closed, flutter open briefly, and I can see that they are deviated to the far right, as though he is looking for something important that has dropped on the floor.

Poor Dan, rumpled and exhausted at the end of his overnight call, has also materialized. "He's not protecting his airway," he says tersely, looking to me.

"We're going to have to tube him," I agree, unzipping my bag. Taking my equipment out, I turn to our nurses. "We're going to have to call a code. Let's get the code cart over here and some more people to help. Page the attending, please." I am deliberately talking slowly, calmly, keeping my voice down, having slipped into my standard emergency personality. I tell myself that it's a strategy to keep everyone else calm, because one more person running around screaming isn't going to help anything, though I know that the main person that I'm aiming to keep calm is myself. But even with this attempt at self-hypnosis, I am not anywhere close to succeeding. I can tell from the way I am fumbling my equipment, the way my hand shakes as I click open the laryngoscope and slip in the endotracheal tube. The voice of one of my old medical school professors plays in my head. *During an arrest, the first set of vital signs you need to take is your own.*

I can't really remember my own wedding, not the way I remember other, less important events. I remember little snippets of it—steaming the wrinkles out of my dress, walking back down the aisle after being pronounced husband and wife, the small taste of wedding cake I got to enjoy before being whisked away by various obligations—but there are huge swaths of the day that are just hazy impressions, like unfocused slide projections on a distant screen. This particular arrest is much the same way. I am intubating the patient, trying to get a set of vital signs, yelling for the Doppler probe. There is a cut, and the next scene is that of a full complement of at least six or seven Anesthesia attendings gathered around the patient, all trying in vain to get more vascular access, to draw blood for labs, to place an arterial line. One or two Anesthesia attendings or residents are grouped on each of Mr. Lozada's four limbs, all making futile passes with their needles, fishing for blood. One attending is placing a central line into the internal jugular vein, diving again and again into Mr. Lozada's thin neck with a huge needle, noting, "This patient is dry as a bone." I remember—and this may be anytime from five to twenty minutes later—finally throwing an arterial line in his left wrist, that column of bright red blood after so many failed attempts as improbable and miraculous as taking a pancake off the griddle and finding a browned, bas relief Virgin Mary looking back at me. "Nice one!" one of my coresidents hoots—he has been fishing around on the opposite arm—but I don't feel nearly as elated. This is *my* patient. Even though I followed the treatment plan of his primary surgeons, I feel like whatever is happening to him right now may, at least in part, be related to something I did, or more probably, *failed* to do, to take care of him. I feel like this whole scene is my fault.

There is another cut in the film, and the next thing I know, Mr. Lozada is being wheeled back into the operating room emergently, bags of blood hanging over his head, transport monitor flashing vital signs that, despite our aggressive resuscitation, look all wrong. I help push him to as far as the door of the operating room but, because I am not wearing a mask or a head cover, cannot step in. Instead, I helplessly watch through the window, the flurry of arms and bags and wires and tubes all narrowly missing one another, that familiar dance of order and chaos.

* * *

I find out later that when Mr. Lozada arrested, his hematocrit was 17. The neurologists, who somehow homed in on the scene like sharks smelling blood in the water, postulated that the patient had had a stroke shortly after being moved to his transport stretcher, though if it followed from a blood clot to the brain or just his low blood count, they were unable to say. It was also unclear *when* exactly his blood count had taken that precipitous drop. Did the bleeding, under control for hours, pick up again after he was jostled onto the transport stretcher that morning? Or had he been slowly bleeding all through the night, and it didn't manifest in his vital signs until things reached a head that morning? What had I done wrong? What should I have done instead? What did I miss?

My attending, looking a little shaken but far more composed than I, has a more philosophical approach. *Sometimes, with very sick patients, these things happen.* And though I know this to be true intellectually, something illogical in me insists that what happened to Mr. Lozada is my fault. I go through the events of the night over and over again, combing for details that I may have missed, the paths not taken. If only I had drawn one more blood sample a few hours earlier, maybe I would have caught something developing. If only I had argued harder with the Vascular Surgery attending, insisting that the patient be transfused, maybe we wouldn't have gotten so far behind. If only I had placed that arterial line sooner. If only I hadn't gone to Grand Rounds. Would any of these things have helped? Would any of these things have saved him?

Residents are by nature egocentric. Not egocentric necessarily in the way of high self-esteem (though there are certainly those among us who make up for the rest), but egocentric in the way that a young child is egocentric, in the sense that everything in the world somehow reflects back to you. It takes time, experience, and probably a certain degree of world-weariness to come to the point where you realize that not everything can be prevented. Not everything is your fault. Sometimes, no amount of caring or earnestness or good intention can stave off a bad outcome, though hopefully, we still try. Hopefully, we never get so jaded that we stop trying.

I'm sure I'll still be thinking, years later, about what I would have done differently if I'd had another chance—of all the codes I've attended, Mr. Lozada's is by far one of the most personal. It was not a code to which I just waltzed in at the critical moment, completed my job, and then walked away. This was *my* code. This was *my* patient.

Mr. Lozada goes into cardiac arrest three more times in the operating room, but he survives long enough to leave the table and is wheeled to the Surgical ICU several hours later in critical condition. His family, initially adamant that everything possible be done to keep him alive, eventually reconsiders in the face of his clinical picture, and care is withdrawn the next day. He dies soon thereafter.

The chance to attend codes is something every young doctor should get, if for no other reason than to experience medicine at its most raw. Though sometimes blurred, there is a distinct line between life and death, and only at a code does a resident get a chance to tread directly on that line. There is nothing like being able to wrench a patient back over that divide, and there is nothing like that feeling that today, someone was trying to die, but *you wouldn't let them.*

That adrenaline, that power, is the stuff that hospital shows and movies are made of. "Breathe!" puffs Anthony Edwards in *ER*, bald pate gleaming. "Don't die on me, man! Breathe!" No one actually makes such exhortations aloud to a coding patient in a real hospital, but inside our heads, that's what we're all thinking.

And yet, after having been to enough codes, one sees the ugly reality of it all. The purple-gray face of the patient after a cardiac arrest. The fecal stink of a patient having lost bowel control in those final moments of life. The glazed, bleary film that develops over a cornea when a patient can no longer blink. Prying open a cold mouth only to encounter an airway full of thick, yellow vomit, filling the space between the vocal cords and seeping down into the lungs. This gritty realness, so distant from the gauzy heroism depicted for the entertainment of laymen, is enough to make good doctors turn their attention toward fields like pathology, radiology, or psychiatry. To be with a person fighting and losing that messy battle against death is closer than most want to be. But going to codes gives you a perspective that you might not otherwise have. To be confronted daily with the proximity of death gives you an amazing appreciation for its inverse.

After my night on call with Mr. Lozada, I stumble home in a daze, looking at but not really seeing the subway cars whizzing by and the New York street traffic narrowly evading pedestrians. *Consider*, I think suddenly in amazement, *all that is happening in hospitals around the city at this very moment, yet outside here in the real world, life goes on as usual.* Here, among people who are healthy, vital, walking down the street on their own two legs, hearts beating strong in their chests, lungs filling on their own with fresh, autumn air, completely unaware of the miracle of it all.

8. A REAL DOCTOR

Leaving the Nest

AFTER WE FINISHED OUR SURGICAL CLERKSHIPS in June of our third year of medical school, our preceptor, an impossibly cool cardiothoracic surgeon named Niloo Edwards, took all four of the students in his rotation group out to a local bar for drinks. We had never been taken out for drinks by an attending before, certainly not a tall, handsome one with a continental accent who rode a motorcycle and dressed in a style I would classify as Urban Safari Chic—and we all tried desperately not to embarrass ourselves. As sheltered medical students apparently incapable of discussing anything else, conversation started with shop talk, devolved into fretting about exams, and then inevitably turned to the subject of residency.

"There's just one thing you need to know about

residency," Dr. Edwards broke in, the glass of his gin and tonic stamping interlinking watery circles on the countertop. "First, there is pain. Then, there is *more* pain. Then you start to *love* the pain."

You would be hard-pressed to find a medical resident who doesn't long to be finished with training. Even the most academic, committed, and self-flagellating person on the planet has to look beyond the scut and the subordination and the nights of endless call to something bigger, something beyond, and see the light at the end of the tunnel that is graduation. Sometimes, it seems like this hope of better things is all there is to keep us going. *Yes, this is miserable,* we tell ourselves, *but above all, it is temporary.*

The strange thing about residency, however, is that you start to develop a sort of Stockholm syndrome once you get close to graduation. Once you start to get a good view outside of those gates and see how vast and endless and *unsupervised* the world beyond residency really is, you start to appreciate for the first time how very reassuring it is to be constantly told what to do. There's something easy and passive and comfortable about being an underling. As a resident, you don't always ask for the advice of your attendings, and you don't always *want* to follow the orders that you are given, but when push comes to shove, if things go wrong, the ultimate responsibility does not fall to you. You can blame yourself for bad outcomes all you want, but in the eyes of the law, it's never really *your* fault.

Once you start nearing completion of the process, the things that once annoyed you about residency start to feel strangely reassuring. There's always someone watching over your every move. The daily rhythm of your day is tedious but familiar. And if you're ever in a bind, or if you don't know what to do, you can always defer to your attending, with the understandable excuse that *hey, you're just a resident.* It's only when you aren't able to use that line anymore that you realize just how nice it was to have a catch-all reason for not always knowing what to do.

Of course, the point of residency is not to make you want to be a resident forever. The point is to teach you enough so that you're prepared for what's next. Yes, the cheap and unflinching slave labor the hospital receives in return is a bonus, but as with raising a child, any residency director will tell you that the time and resources devoted to training a good resident far outstrip that which the resident herself has put in. Like children, we start residency bald and defenseless, grow up chafing and occasionally rebelling against authority, and finally mellow and start to appreciate the comforts of our sheltered home.

And then just when we start to get comfortable, they kick us out into the world.

* * *

"So what do you want to be when you grow up?"

It is my third and final year of Anesthesia residency, and one of my classmates is asking me about my plans for the future. It seems that in one way or another, everyone else in my class is falling into line. Some of my classmates, of course, are looking for jobs, excited about the prospect of finally finishing training and leaving the scutmonkey era behind, not to mention the appeal of working fewer hours for more money. However, a sizeable portion of my class has also decided to pursue fellowship training in a specialized area of anesthesia (for example, pediatric anesthesia or critical care), in the interest of having a little more training under their belts before being released into the wild.

I have heard of fellowship training being called "a $300,000 mistake," referring to the year of lost income during a fellowship year, in a job field where, with a few exceptions, fellowships are not essential or required. However, I can also easily see the appeal of prolonging training for another year. Another year in the greenhouse, another year with a safety net. *If I spend another year in training, maybe* then *I'll actually feel ready to be a real doctor.*

While I have certainly reached the point in my residency where I feel ready to work independently—I am excited at the prospect of doing cases entirely on my own, and catch myself feeling annoyed or smothered when attendings come to check in too often—I also realize that much of this adolescent hunger for autonomy is couched in the underlying knowledge that I always have someone to bail me out if I get in over my head. There is a distinct line between being allowed to work independently and being hung out to dry. Like a teenager, I want to distance myself from my parents, walk ten feet in front of them down the sidewalk, be viewed as my own person, but I also know that I will never really be left alone in the ruins of my own mistakes.

So for lack of any better plan, I decide to do a fellowship. I apply for and am accepted to Columbia's one-year fellowship in Regional Anesthesia, a procedure-based specialty offshoot based on techniques of peripheral nerve blockade and acute pain management. And so I have signed on to extend my training for another year. In one sense it is something of a relief to finally have committed to a course of action, and a respectable course at that, with an academic rationale to hide behind. But as the euphoria wears off and the reality sets in, I sense that there is also another feeling underlying, one decidedly more complex. I keep thinking of agoraphobics, of shut-ins, of thirty-year-old men still living in their parents' basements. In some ways, I feel like I have decided to stick around for another year because the prospect of dealing with the outside world is too daunting, and I'm afraid to leave.

Rerouted

And then, a few weeks after I accepted my fellowship position at Columbia, Joe gets some news.

For the past two years, Joe has been in the long, drawn-out process of applying for a fellowship in oculoplastics, a little-known and extremely competitive offshoot of ophthalmology dealing with corrective and reconstructive surgery of the soft tissues around the eye. These fellowship spots are few and far between, most of the available programs taking only one fellow every other year. Joe applied across the country, but of course, there are no guarantees. We are assessing our choices, I planning my next step, when we hear from an oculoplastics program in Atlanta, run through Emory University Hospital. They would be delighted, they tell us, to have Joe join them to start his fellowship training in oculoplastics, starting this summer. *In Atlanta.*

To put it mildly, this complicates things somewhat.

On one hand, having choices is almost always a good thing. And Joe's match, after so many years of work and months of frustration, is undeniably great news. All told, with the day-to-day toil of residency, the pressure to do research and publish, and a month of travel on the interview trail, this process of applying for a fellowship has entailed a substantial amount of work, complicated by the sort of weary cynicism that accompanies any large investment for which one is not assured any results at all.

But while hearing about Joe's fellowship is great news on one front, it evokes in both of us an emotion that falls just short of happiness. Because by accepting this fellowship spot and relocating to Atlanta, we are basically giving up absolutely everything else. Obviously, I had been planning to do a fellowship at Columbia the following year, and I will have to give that up. My parents live in New York, and we will have to move away from them. We have housing, childcare, a network of people up here, and when we move, we will be saying good-bye to it all.

From that point of view, the scales look a little uneven. And this imbalance causes the feminist inside me to cringe.

Because Joe's fellowship is so competitive, we agreed early on in the process that if he were fortunate enough to match into a program, wherever it might be, we would all pick up and move there without question for the two years it would take him to complete his training. After all, a good oculoplastics fellowship is a rare bird indeed. You just don't turn down a good position like that, because another one may never come along.

I have to admit, however, in the moments of self-pity following the news from Atlanta, that I feel a certain 1970s Hillary Clinton–esque martyrdom in the whole decision. What about *my* career, *my* training? Why should we automatically move to accommodate *Joe's* career? Is there a certain latent sexism on both our parts to presume that this should happen? Why move for him and give up everything else, as opposed to staying for me?

Of course, nothing is quite so black and white. Despite my initial reflexive reaction to uprooting our entire lives for this fellowship, I can see that it's not *just* about Joe's career. Compared with some of the other fellowships that we've looked at, this one offers a better quality of life for its fellows, allowing him to spend more time with me and Cal, have shorter hours, less intense call. And after he's done with his fellowship, he will hopefully also be able to have a better lifestyle overall. Again, better hours, better income, and more importantly, he will be happy doing the kind of surgery and practicing the kind of medicine that he enjoys.

I have, several times in the past, told Joe to just forget about any further training in plastics, to just finish out his training in general ophthalmology, work part-time, and stay home with Cal the rest of the week. *It would be win-win,* I told him, only partially kidding. (OK, so maybe I wasn't kidding at all.) *I would have the peace of mind knowing that Cal's spending time with a parent, and I would be more than happy to work full-time and bring home the bacon.*

But for Joe, this has never been a serious option—for him, it's never been about the income so much as the *work.* While the need to put food on the table is a real one, in the end, he needs to be able to do the kind of work that makes him happy. He has decided that he wants to do plastics. He would thrive doing plastics. And now he has a chance to get the specialized training that he needs.

And so it is settled—really, in the end, there is never any question, and it amounts to not so much of a subversion of my own plans as a global plan for our family and what's best for all of us. I will not be doing the fellowship at Columbia. We are moving to Atlanta. And I will need to find a job. It is time to grow up after all. It's time to deal with what comes next.

"You'll stay in academics," Craig predicts, the same classmate who asked me before what I wanted to be when I grew up. "I can see it."

"Oh really?" I consider this. "Why do you say that?"

"Because," he smirks, his default facial expression, "that's your personality. You're a woman, a mommy type. You just want to take care of people and make people happy."

I stand up, draining my can of soda, and prepare to return to the operating room. "I'm already a doctor, Craig," I say. "Regardless of being a mom or not, I think that wanting to take care of people is part of the package."

* * *

"I'm sure you'll be able to find a mommy job."

"What did you say? A *funny* job?" I am sitting with one of my attendings in the Anesthesia conference room, where we are both eating lunch—it is loud, so I can't quite hear what he is saying. He is one of the younger attendings in the Pediatrics Department, and spent some time in "the real world" before taking an academic position at Columbia. I have specifically been asking him about the job market out there, having no idea what said job market looks like or how I am supposed to break into it. In fact, as I brush up my curriculum vitae, I realize that, outside of residency, I have never *had* a real job. I have had summer positions or worked in research, but most of the work I've done, if I've been paid for it at all, has been more of the "$600 stipend for the summer" variety. So here I am, this adult woman, almost in her thirties but apparently only just on the brink of adulthood, who has no idea how to support herself.

"A *mommy* job," he repeats, a little bit louder. "You'll have no problem finding a job like that." I have just been asking him about the availability, so far as he is aware, of jobs that would offer me the ability to work part-time, or to avoid working nights. As a fellow in Atlanta, Joe will be on call every night for two years straight, and I want to try as much as I can to have at least one parent at home in the evenings.

"Well, why is that a *mommy* job?" I respond snappishly, my feminist guard dog springing reflexively into action. "Don't *fathers* want to spend time with their kids too? Don't fathers in medicine ever consider taking part-time or no-call jobs in order to smooth out issues with childcare or family life?" But all I need to do is take in the blank, silent stare of everyone observing this exchange and to reflect on my own experiences to realize that no, they do not. *All* jobs in medicine are "daddy jobs."

And really, why am I even offended? Isn't it *true*? After all, I *am* a mother, and like most working mothers, I am looking for a job that would allow me to balance the needs of my child with the needs of my career. What is so wrong with *that*? Why would I react as though I am being accused of laziness, of requesting special favors? Is it just because of this desire to show that I am up for any challenge? To prove that there's nothing outside of the hospital that can interfere with what I'm doing inside of it? To squelch any notion that women in medicine may have different concerns than men? Or is it just the diminutive "mommy job" designation that has me up in arms? What is it exactly that is pushing my buttons anyway?

"But I see what you're saying," I finally concede diplomatically, trying to smooth over my previous outburst. "That *is* the kind of position that I'm looking for. I just...I'm just looking for a way to advance my career without totally neglecting my kid, you know? It's hard. But at least there are jobs like that out there. Thanks for the tips."

"I think," one of my other coresidents, Adam, offers seriously, helpfully, "that you shouldn't try to get a job at *all.* I think you should just take two years off and have another baby or two."

With this lofty set of expectations, I have to wonder, would anyone dare to offer me, a female physician in her childbearing years, a job at all?

How to Find a Job in Anesthesia, Theater of the Mind Edition

MICHELLE: I am graduating from Anesthesia residency, and I need a job.

HOSPITAL ADMINISTRATOR: And why should we give you a job?

MICHELLE: Because I need one. And also, I am awesome.

HOSPITAL ADMINISTRATOR: Excellent, Doctor. You can start in July, with full benefits and a parking space in the physicians' lot. Would this giant wad of cash be sufficient to seal the deal?

MICHELLE: Yes, please.

(Fin)

How to Find a Job in Anesthesia, Reality Edition

MICHELLE: I am graduating from Anesthesia residency, and I need a job.

(Crickets.)

MICHELLE: I need a job. Hello? Is anyone listening?

(Silence. In the distance, a wolf howls.)

MICHELLE: Will administer anesthesia for food!

BYSTANDER: Hey, have you tried looking at the job postings on any of those medical recruiter sites? Or maybe you should try calling some of the hospitals in Atlanta, near where you're going to be living. You know, see if there are any job openings with the Anesthesia Department.

MICHELLE: I have to do *what* now?

(Fin)

No, Really, How to Find a Job in Anesthesia

STEP 1: Pull up a map of Atlanta on Google. Look for all the little pink buildings on the map, which indicate the hospitals. Write down all the names of the hospitals in the metro area.

STEP 2: Wonder why, looking at this same map, every other street in Atlanta appears to have the word "Peachtree" in it. Peachtree Avenue. Peachtree

Road. Peachtree Plaza. Peachtree Industrial Boulevard. *This* isn't going to be confusing.

STEP 3: Again, with the aid of Google, look up each hospital's website in an attempt to figure out exactly which hospitals are affiliated with each other and what anesthesia group services which hospital. This is somewhat more difficult to figure out than it might appear at first glance, because, despite the crucial importance of anesthesia in many aspects of patient care, it remains something of a behind-the-scenes, "pay no attention to the man behind the curtain" specialty, and as such, information about the Anesthesia Department is not exactly a prominent feature on any hospital's homepage.

STEP 4: Dial what you think is the phone number for the Anesthesia Department of the first hospital.

STEP 5: Wrong number.

STEP 6: Disconnected number.

STEP 7: High-pitched squealing and electronic trills indicates that you probably just called a fax machine.

STEP 8: Finally get through to a real, presumably live, human being. "Hi, my name is [Michelle Au],* I'm a third-year Anesthesia resident at Columbia Presbyterian Hospital in New York, and I was wondering if there were any potential job openings with your group and whether or not I could send you my CV." A secretary on the other end

---

*Feel free to insert your name here to use as a template for your own job search. You're welcome.

has no idea, but is willing to accept your CV to "pass along." It is not clear who exactly she is going to pass it along *to*, nor whether there is an actual job to which you are applying, but you readily take her e-mail address and beam a copy of your credentials out into the void.

STEP 9: Repeat Steps 4 through 8 for each subsequent hospital on your list. Don't forget to factor in time for futile head-banging and grumbled obscenities directed at no one in particular, which, while not actually helpful in finding a job, tend to quiet the yammering voices in your head saying that there is simply no way you are ready yet to go out into the real world and pretend be a real doctor.

STEP 10: The garden is seeded. Now to let the job offers come rolling in! Aaaand...*go*!

STEP 11: Go!

STEP 12: Hmm. Maybe your phone is broken. Nope, seems to be working.

STEP 13: Maybe your e-mail account is broken too. True, you have received three e-mails from Nigerian aristocracy so far today, promising to wire you a sum in excess of fifteen million dollars in exchange for your social security number and bank account access, but curiously no word from any of the hospitals that you applied to.

STEP 14: Check your spam folder, just in case.

STEP 15: Quietly start tearing your hair out.

STEP 16: Finally, start hearing back from some of the anesthesia groups to which you applied. While most seem leery about even confirming that they have a definite job opening available, they are all excessively gracious (a common trait in people from the South, you will soon find) and are more than happy to set up an interview so that you can visit the hospitals, meet the partners, and see their practice in action. If it seems like a good fit, they will keep you in mind in the event a position does open up.

STEP 17: You have a series of interviews set up. Dig out your suit and heels (only slightly dusty having been in the closet for the last five years, since the last time you had to wear them for residency interviews) and inspect them for more egregious signs of age. True, there is a small moth hole in the lining of the jacket and some unraveling along one of the inside seams, but as long as you keep your jacket buttoned at all times, no one will be the wiser! Print out extra copies of CV to carry around and dispense like headshots at an audition. Grab tacky-looking fake leather portfolio embossed with medical school insignia to tote it all around with you. And smile! With *confidence*! Now all you have to do is go to the interview and convince them all that you're an actual competent doctor and capable of performing as such.

STEP 18: Complete the task of tearing your hair out. There are a few wisps in the back that you missed the first time around.

* * *

At the point in your medical career where you are looking for your first job, idealism and practicality inevitably collide. Medical students and even residents live to some extent in a protected bubble of jejune sentiment, and this is for a number of reasons. First, as trainees, we are relatively protected—from liability, from responsibility, from the financial bottom line of the medical care we provide. Secondly, though wide-eyed wonder gives way to a more grounded set of real-world concerns, doctors coming out of training are still relatively naïve when it comes to the interface of medicine and business. That is, while medicine is a calling, and while many doctors love what they do, it is still a job, and the same concerns of any job still apply.

In other words: I will be getting paid, right? I've been in various stages of medical training for a total of nine years now, living the impecunious life of the indentured servant, and though I'm still too embarrassed to say it out loud to anyone, the truth of the matter is that I *need* to get paid. Since Joe will still be in training for the next two years, the pressure is on me to be the breadwinner for our family, and I need to find a job that can support all of us.

The other problem is that, again, since Joe will still be in training, the burden *also* falls to me to be flexible enough in my job schedule so that I can take care of things at home if Joe gets called in the middle of the night for emergencies. Because as the sole oculoplastics fellow for the department, he will be on call all night, *every* night, for two years straight, and as such there are no guarantees that he will ever be home at any given hour, basically ever. This fact introduces the central point of conflict into our lives, one which will probably stress our marriage the most in the years to come. In essence, I feel as though I am being asked to do *everything*.

"You know, *classically*, there's a division of labor on these matters," I fume. "Usually the breadwinner of the household is not *also* expected to be the primary homemaker. This situation puts a lot of stress on me, you know. And what kind of a bum deal is this, anyway? I do *everything* while you make *no* money *and* are never home? Does that seem equitable to you?" To his credit, Joe realizes that there is no good answer to this question, nor should he even try to come up with one. Though perhaps feigning sleep was a touch of theatrics he should have skipped.

So what is obvious now is that I will need a full-time job, though I also need a job that allows me to come home every evening without any overnight shifts. In the real world, this is simply known as "a job"; however, in medicine, the requirement to not be at work at, say, three o'clock in the morning, is something that needs to be explicitly spelled out. There's no way Joe and I could swing it otherwise. While childproof locks and remote surveillance technology have no doubt progressed light-years in the past few decades, until the development of a twenty-four-hour robotic nanny, there's simply no way we could manage the need for late-night childcare if both Joe and I were both on-call overnight and called in simultaneously.

The first practice for which I have interviewed seems most receptive to the idea of a five-day-a-week position, but warns that this is somewhat new territory for them and that further discussion would need to take place before such could be offered. At my second job interview, I don't even bother to push the issue, as the employee handbook I have been given to read beforehand explicitly states that with the exception of employees pushing retirement age and who have been with the department for more than fifteen years, *everyone* must take call, no exceptions whatsoever. And the third practice I visit somewhat apologetically notes that part of the reason they are even *looking* for a new hire in the first place is to find another person with whom to split the overnight call duty, because they are all working too many nights as it is and are damn tired of it.

Despite the reasonable nature of my need to find a call-free job, what I find during my interviews is that I feel surprisingly guilty and abashed to even ask for such a position, as though I am somehow compromising my professional integrity by bringing up my responsibilities at home. The guilt is internalized, but it doesn't come from me, exactly. While such a position would unequivocally be the best for me and my family, and would still probably entail me working around fifty hours per week, there is this notion in medicine (most probably passed down from The Days of the Giants, the era when the ability to sacrifice everything in the name of medicine was considered a doctor's greatest virtue) that younger doctors who elect to place lifestyle ahead of professional pursuits are, for lack of a better term, *total pansies*. Older doctors often decry the erosion of work ethic with each subsequent generation of residents, and even within my own group of residents, I have groused privately about the diligence and stamina of some of our juniors, some of whom seem to have come into medicine with a completely different sense of what would be expected of them than what I had been raised with. Given that, I can't imagine what the doctors of the Golden Age would think about *my* professional goals, to have my nights and weekends to spend at home taking care of my son. While I don't agree with them that the only good doctor is the one who lives, breathes, eats, and sleeps medicine (though sleeping only four hours a night, mind you), I do feel somehow that I am betraying those ideals by opting for the alternative.

It is a central theme of struggle for working mothers, though I daresay it is particularly acute for doctors who are mothers, as the culture of medicine has lagged behind some of the more family-friendly models seen in other fields. One truly feels that she cannot win. On one hand, we are compromising our medical careers, plotting half-assed trajectories working what are perceived as subprime careers, to the point that it has been argued that it is less fiscally responsible to train a female medical student than a male one, for the return received on investment. And on the other end, both the internal and societal guilt and pressure on the working mother are already well documented. We are told early on that medicine is our calling, our focus, but how can our own families not mandate at least as much of our attention? It is no wonder that we are unsure how to act, how to present ourselves, and how others dealing with these issues feel much of the same pressure to ignore the white elephant in the room.

At one of my job interviews, I am spending time chatting with one of the partners on his lunch break; he is a jovial, middle-aged male anesthesiologist who I could imagine in his college days with Greek letters written on his chest in greasepaint, balancing upside-down over a keg. We are having a pleasant conversation, talking about this and that, not even about the job or anesthesia or medicine in particular, when he casually asks, "So, how old is your son?"

I start to answer this perfectly natural question, when he leans forward and stops me midsentence. "Oops. Wait, I don't think I'm allowed to ask you that."

* * *

I get the job that I want.

It is with the first practice at which I interviewed, the one that was most receptive to the idea of having some flexibility with respect to me taking night call. The partners have met among themselves and have agreed to offer me what basically amounts to a Monday-through-Friday job, with no night call, no weekends, no holidays. The pay is decent and the benefits are excellent. If I'm interested, I can start this summer.

I believe it is accurate to say that I cannot sign this job contract fast enough.

The anxiety about finding a job now on the side-lines (aside from the occasional neurotic twinge that they might change their minds for some reason and rescind the offer—I had the same flashes of neurosis after I got accepted to medical school), I can concentrate all my anxiety on what it actually means to *have* a job.

Of all the jobs for which I interviewed, the one that I accepted is undoubtedly the most challenging, and the one for which I currently feel the most unprepared. I will regularly be doing anesthesia for open-heart surgery, with which I had fair experience during residency but do not quite feel ready to do on my own. The facilities are huge, the patient population sick, the average acuity of care very high. On my tour of the hospital on interview day, I peeked out the window of the emergency room and saw an open concrete flat, something like a basketball field. "Oh," said the anesthesiologist showing me around, noting my questioning expression, "that's our helipad. They fly patients in here from around the state for cardiac surgery."

Of course, I addressed some of these concerns with the group when I interviewed, not wanting to sell them a false bill about my abilities and having particular concerns about being a fresh graduate put in what appeared to me to be a fast-paced, high-demand practice. Overall, they were unconcerned about what I perceive to be my inexperience, trusted in my training, and responded that they had traditionally hired many people straight out of residency or fellowship, and that I should not think of this job as being thrown to the wolves but rather as a continuation of my education and professional development. "Sure, it's a little scary at first," said one of the younger anesthesiologists in the group, "but you do a lot of learning on the job, and if you ever need help with something, you can always just call someone. Everyone's been through it. Everyone's here to help." I flashed back to my first month of Anesthesia residency, when I could not believe that I was being left alone with my patient on a ventilator and the thousand things that could go wrong. "Just call me if you need me," my attending would always tell me. "But use your judgment. You know more than you think you do."

Probably there were easier jobs for me to take straight out of residency—maybe a nice softball office-based anesthesia job like sedation at an endoscopy center, or doing anesthesia for small, outpatient surgical procedures. The transition would be easier certainly, and at this point I could do cases like that on my own without a second thought. But then, what would be the fun of *that*? What would be the fun in spending all those years in training, doing anesthesia for neurosurgery, organ transplants, open-heart cases, only to take a job in which I wouldn't be able to use any of these skills? If anything, fresh from residency and flush with academic idealism, *this* was the time to push myself, to take a job that I felt was a little beyond me, as long as there were mechanisms in place to ask for help if I needed it, to learn from those more experienced than I before becoming more experienced myself. Isn't this what my entire medical training has been up through this point, after all? Pushing the limits a little at a time, never letting myself get too comfortable with my knowledge and my skills, always looking to do something that's a little bit out of my reach, and then doing it again and again, until finally, unbelievably, it's second nature?

I take the job. And charged with fresh purpose, I get out my textbooks and resume studying—this time not for an exam, but for my new job. I am graduating from residency in sixteen weeks and it is incomprehensible and frankly a little overwhelming how much I still have to learn.

* * *

Let me talk for a moment about fear.

As with most things in medicine, fear can be broken up into two categories, acute and chronic. Acute fear can come out of nowhere, like a sudden cardiac arrest, or the thunderclap headache heralding rupture of a cerebral aneurysm. One moment you're sitting down at the nursing station, checking labs or writing notes or any number of mundane and yet endless tasks which consume probably 75 percent of a resident's time. And the next moment you're getting paged stat to one of the operating rooms on Labor and Delivery, where, upon your rushing through the door, a nurse thrusts a grayish purple, flaccid, and completely unresponsive newborn into your arms, still slick with greenish brown meconium, the imprint of the giant metal forceps from delivery still visible over each ear. *Oh shit.* Or being called emergently into a patient's room early one evening, where you find her disoriented, wearing only a pair of underwear, the front of her gown wide open, copiously vomiting what looks like a gallon of congealed blood onto the floor next to her bed. *Oh shit.* Or arriving at a stat intubation up on one of the patient floors, to find a cachectic patient teetering on the edge of respiratory failure, a patient who, you're told, has had a series of strokes that render him unable to open his mouth, and some unfortunate head and neck tumors that are likely critically compressing his trachea. Once again, *oh shit.*

Acute fear is visceral, mind numbing, time warping, and the closest I can come to describing it is being hurled headfirst into a plunge pool filled with ice water. And the instinct, at any level of training, is immediate and reflexive, a fight-or-flight response. *I know that I'm responsible for taking care of this patient, and now I have to figure out what I'm going to do,* the rational mind says. However, underneath the rational, upon being exposed to such horror, seeing things that no one in their right mind would ever want to see, the overpowering instinct is, simply, to run away.

Everyone has a handful of acute-fear stories, and we share them readily, because in a weird way, *having* been so scared and weathering the storm is sort of affirming. All you need to do is get a couple of doctors around a table, give them a few beers, and the next thing you know, everyone is coming out with their favorite *oh shit* stories, trading them around like baseball cards. One of my personal favorites (if it's not macabre to call it that) involves a liver transplant for which I was the resident anesthesiologist, where, in the middle of the case, I heard a continuous splattering sound, like water hitting tile, and when I looked under the operating table, I saw blood running, literally like out of a faucet, from the abdomen of the patient and cascading in rivers onto the floor. The nurses, meanwhile, were frantically running around the room, spreading blankets under our feet so that we wouldn't slip, blankets that were becoming soaked basically as fast as they could lay them down. Acute fear is *interesting*, it is *exciting*, and for the most part, we are open about it because it usually implies some catastrophic event separate from ourselves that we cannot control, leaving us for the most part blameless.

And then there's chronic fear. Chronic fear is of the slow, simmering variety, built up over days or weeks or even years, and as such factors in much more time for second-guessing and rationalization. There are many variations of chronic fear, found at many different stages of one's medical career, but it all boils down to approximately the same thing. *I am scared because I don't know if I can do this. I don't feel like I have the skills. I don't want to hurt my patients with my mistakes. I don't know if I have been adequately trained to do this, I don't feel ready, yet here I am.*

Doctors don't talk as much about chronic fear.

Though I don't doubt that a doctor's chronic-fear level has an inversely proportional relationship to the number of his or her years in practice, probably most physicians feel some level of chronic fear at some point. As a resident, I am well acquainted with the phenomenon, but I see fleeting glimpses of it in my attendings too, when pushed into situations outside of their comfort zones. Everyone feels inadequacy at some point, because even the best physicians cannot possibly be expert in everything.

Obviously, the reason that we don't talk much about chronic fear is that no one wants to admit that they've even entertained the notion that we may not be good enough to do our jobs. Part of it stems from the extremely high expectations that society has for its doctors, and that doctors have for themselves. *I'm smart. I went to medical school. I've been in training for years. I've jumped over every hurdle, worked hard, people seem to trust me, rely on me to know what I'm doing. So how do I deal with the nagging feeling that I'm just not quite ready?* Chronic fear, basically, is just not *cool*. So we don't talk about it. We continue to work hard, amplify our experience and confidence, and hope that soon enough, our self-image will catch up to the outward image that we project.

I think that fear can sometimes be a good thing, though. Obviously, maladaptive fear is not—I think that curling in a ball in the corner of the OR, rocking back and forth while keening about one's perceived inadequacy, has very little therapeutic value for our patients *or* for ourselves—but I think that every physician should always be able to feel a small amount of fear. Fear is a stimulus to be better. Fear protects you from hubris. Fear is a guard against complacency. And frankly, I think that fear is a form of respect—to the patient, to the practice of medicine, to the knowledge that despite best intentions, things don't always go as planned.

We are entrusted with the lives of our patients every day. In anesthesia, we essentially take the entire being of the patient into our hands, shutting down their consciousness, taking over the function of their lungs, their hearts, the blood flow to their organs, the very delivery of oxygen that keeps each cell of their body alive. And every day, we tell our patients that at the end of it all, we will return their bodies to them, undamaged or in some cases even improved, and patients for the most part trust that we will do just that. This is the job that we do each day. And every mistake we make while caring for our patients, every tactical misstep or error in judgment, feels like a breach of that trust. Fear? How can we *not* be afraid? The day you sit back and think that you're infallible is the day your clinical instincts are gone.

In other words, if you don't admit to being scared sometimes, you're an asshole.

* * *

My last day of residency is Sunday, June 29, 2008, taking home call for cardiothoracic anesthesia, and I have to admit, I am hoping for a softball.

I figure I will get called in for *something* at the very least, but maybe something small, like a washout of a wound, or maybe a chest closure. Our moving van is scheduled to come early the next morning, so I requested this Sunday on call to give myself the chance to actually be physically present the next day, as burly men will be descending on our home, wrapping and packing everything we own for our move to Atlanta. I am hoping, perhaps naïvely, that I might even get a chance to finish some packing later this evening. A quiet end to my residency, while anticlimactic, would certainly be convenient.

I already know from the night before that they have scheduled a BiVAD—essentially, the placement of a mechanical ventricular assist device, often used in failing hearts as a bridge to transplant—to start at 8:00 a.m. So I am already prepared to go in for that case, which will undoubtedly take a good couple of hours, at least until the afternoon. But there is always the possibility that the service will be quiet after that. There is nothing else looking ominous up in the CTICU. The OR desk has a blank slate otherwise, as far as they are concerned. I say nothing to jinx myself, but inside my shoes, my toes are crossed.

The BiVAD is going smoothly, patient doing well, when we get word that the thoracic surgeons have just booked a double-lung transplant. Then, moments later, further word that the cardiac team has also just booked a heart transplant. Same donor, two different patients. And that, as they say, is the ballgame.

Once my attending and I realize that the whole day is basically written off, I actually start to enjoy myself. "Going out with a bang!" I keep saying for the rest of the day. My attending is not *quite* so happy at how the cards have fallen, but I think he is pleased enough that this is my last day of residency. "Why?" I joke. "Because I'm *leaving*, and you'll never have to put up with me again?"

"No," he answers, "because you're basically an attending, and so I can leave you alone to manage things." He turns to the surgeons, the perfusionists running the heart-lung bypass machine, anyone who will listen. "Hey, guys, in about eight hours, she's going to be an attending!" Everyone cheers, hooting or shouting *congratulations*, and I thank them, embarrassed and hoping that I am actually ready for all this.

There is a point, I believe, where we are running four cardiac surgery rooms at once. There is one more case that gets rushed in while I am still in with the BiVAD—a post-op bleeder that, thankfully, one of the second-year residents handles. The day has degenerated from routine to borderline chaotic. Fortunately, the general surgery add-on schedule is virtually empty, which allows the general anesthesia call team to pitch in, second-year residents teeing up rooms to start and occasionally helping to get cases under way. We even enlist the help of two of our first-year residents (at least, they are still first-years for the next two days) to help finish a case as the surgeons are closing the patient's chest, transfusing blood products, and running blood gases as I run next door to start the heart transplant. Neither of them have done their cardiothoracic rotations yet, and as I sign out to them and explain the rainbow display of monitoring, warning them what to watch out for before sprinting to the OR next door, I see their hubcap-sized eyes floating over their masks and give them this empty comfort: "Don't worry, you guys are going to be fine." I remember how many times I've been told that during my own training, when I've been put in situations that I felt were completely beyond me, and how meaningless that seemed—"What do you mean I'm going to be *fine*? How about the fact that I don't know what I'm doing? What's going to happen to the patient?"—and yet, it is. Fine, that is. The attending pops in and out of the room until the last of the dressings are on, the second-year residents troubleshoot, and the patient makes it up to the ICU a few hours later, humming VADs in tow.

How fitting, really, to do a heart transplant as your last case of residency. Much like the process of medical training, an organ transplant takes the ordinary and transposes it into extraordinary circumstances—in this case, taking the heart of a freshly deceased patient and having it work in the body of a patient who still might be saved. The recipient this day is a fifty-seven-year-old man with dilated cardiomyopathy—he has a sick and dying heart that did not beat so much as feebly tremble, barely moving enough blood through his body to keep his organs alive. The sight is quite impressive really, once the patient is anesthetized and the sternum sawed open to reveal the chest cavity underneath. The patient's old heart is huge, congested, an angry and mottled purplish mass that looks more like a dead thing in a butcher's window than anything else. We work together to get the patient onto cardiopulmonary bypass, the surgeons snip the old heart out, and suddenly the chest cavity is huge, empty, a yawning expanse waiting to be filled.

For surgery scheduling, there are usually what we call a "send time" and a "cut time," the *send* indicating the time that the patient should be physically wheeled into the OR, and the *cut*, after induction of anesthesia and placement of all the necessary monitoring and lines, the projected time that the surgeons will be making their first incision. In organ transplants, this is all rigorously timed to coincide with the trajectory of the harvested organ—when they clamp the old heart from the donor, how long it will take them to drive (or in this case, fly) back from the harvest site, when they think the organ will be physically arriving at the hospital. All this is designed to minimize what is called the "ischemic time" of the harvested organ, which is the amount of time that the organ needs to be on ice. Basically, the shorter the ischemic time, the better the new heart will perform.

However, as with anything in the hospital, the timing is not as precise as planned, and so after we go on bypass, after the old heart is out, there is some stalling. During the wait, which seems interminable after all the rush, we exchange stories of transplants past, one in particular in which a member of the harvest team grabbed the Playmate cooler with the organ, jumped out of the ambulance, and simply ran across the George Washington Bridge as fast as he could to the hospital rather than wait for the traffic to clear. We laugh at this image for a little while, relishing how fucking *cool* it would be to be able to tell the family offhandedly afterward that *yes, that was me, I didn't want to keep you all waiting, so I ran your wife's heart across the bridge.*

Finally, with some fanfare, the new heart for our patient arrives, about twenty-five minutes later than predicted. The harvest team, we gather, had been stuck in some traffic. The heart is double-bagged and floating in a slurry of ice, looking small and cold and waxy. The surgeons peer at it intently, turning it over in their hands, occasionally trimming away small pieces in preparation for the anastomosis.

As new connections are made, the patient, who has been cooled down for his run on bypass, is gradually allowed to warm up, and with him warms his new heart. It twitches irregularly at first, then starts to beat. Its stiff, claylike appearance melts away as the heart fills with the patient's blood, and it blooms pink, then bright red. It needs to be shocked once, twice, with internal defibrillation paddles, and the connections are inspected, checked for leaks at the suture lines, but by the time the surgeons start to close the sternum, the heart is beating vigorously, snappily, fairly jumping out of the chest like healthy hearts do. The heart looks like it knows what it is doing. As though it has known what it was supposed to do all along.

When the sternum is wired shut, the skin closed, the final dressing taped on, and the surgical drapes are down, I bundle up the patient, ready him for transport, and, while manually squeezing oxygen into his lungs and pushing drugs into his veins, bring him to the ICU, where a team of nurses fall on him ravenously, connecting him to their monitors and chiding me good-naturedly about the tangled disarray of my IV tubing. "Spaghetti!" one nurse chortles, lifting up a particularly knotty segment—despite my best efforts at order, entropy wins again—and though it is late and though I have heard this joke hundreds of times before, I smile.

The patient is doing well. His heart is strong, his blood pressure is stable, and the bleeding issuing forth from the tubes in his chest at this point is minimal. The surgeons have done a good job. *I* have done a good job. The patient and his new heart too are doing their part, and as we watch, they are picking up the work where we left off. Around me, I hear the beeping of monitors, the hiss of ventilators, and the alarms going off in the rooms of patients who have not been as lucky.

As I leave the hospital just past midnight on my last day of residency, exiting onto the busy intersection of 168th Street and Fort Washington Avenue, it occurs to me what I have just done for the last time. It seems surreal. I expected my final moments of residency to be a distinct anticlimax, something a little like Christmas as a child, an event that you talk about and dream about and look forward to all year, only to sit in your pine needle–littered living room on December 26 thinking to yourself, That's *it*? I remember graduating from med school, expecting some sort of revelatory transformation, some sort of dawning wisdom and air of expertise, and finding that the fact of graduation itself endowed me with none of those things.

The feeling I have now is different. I can't quite pinpoint why, but it's different. There's a sense of *rightness* to it all, as though, looking through a telescope at the past five years condensed—all the long hours, the late nights, the humbling and often humiliating lessons, the tragedies only intermittently punctuated by small, imperceptible triumphs—it has all been leading perfectly up to this. It is a huge moment. It is a completely ordinary moment. Just as it should be.

I think back on the past nine years I have spent in training, all the people, all the separate, disconnected stories that, while individually only amounting to amusing anecdotes or small points of interest, now add up to something bigger. It occurs to me that my clinical experience is simply a sum of all these stories, an uneven course to be sure, like a chain of islands in an archipelago, and cohesive only in retrospect, with the realization that it is the culmination of these stories that has shaped me into the doctor I have become, will continue to shape me into the doctor I want to be. And in the years and decades ahead, there will always be more patients, more emergencies, more losses and gains. There will be more stories, and always more lessons to learn from them.

Diamonds are simple carbon molecules, created under high pressure. And medical residents are just ordinary people growing up and learning who they want to be under the most extraordinary of circumstances. After the relative shelter of medical school, there comes that moment to sink or swim. These are not everyday demands that are made of us. All people make mistakes, especially those young and inexperienced in new roles, but when residents make mistakes, people can die. We worry that we may not be ready for the responsibility, and we are scared because we know that ready or not, it doesn't matter. And all of us, one by one, step up.

We learn how to take care of our patients. We

learn how to take care of each other, both in- and outside of the hospital. Sometimes we fail, and sometimes unavoidable bad things happen for which we blame ourselves. But sometimes we succeed, in small ways, and occasionally in spectacular ways. We do things we never thought we'd be able to do. We grow into our white coats. We learn how to be the doctors that our patients need us to be, without losing the essential humanity that brought us here in the first place. And above all, we keep our eye on what's important.

I hail a cab, an indulgence I save for nights on call, climb in, and give the cabbie my home address. It is late, and I hope to get home in time to get a few hours of sleep. Our moving van is set to arrive at 9:00 a.m.

"You're a doctor?" the cabbie asks some minutes into our trip.

"Yes," I answer, and leave it at that. You can never tell what people will follow up with when they find out you're in medicine—I have had no shortage of total strangers who try to get me to spot-diagnose the causes of their various ailments, ranging from recalcitrant rashes to troubling bouts of excessive flatulence—so over the years I've learned that it's best not to volunteer personal information beyond what is asked.

"One of the best doctors in New York, huh?" he says, with a conspiratorial smile.

"Oh, I really doubt that," I say. Then I add, "But I try to be."

"You work at the best *hospital* in New York," the

cabbie continues, "so then you are one of the *best*. That's what I mean."

"Believe me, there are *plenty* of doctors out there better and more experienced than me," I tell him, "but how about I say that I'll keep working at it?" We both smile, and fall into a companionable silence, he listening to a Pakistani talk show on the radio, I looking out the window at the darkened Queens skyline across the East River, as we speed down the FDR Drive toward my apartment, where my husband and son are asleep, waiting for me to get home.

ACKNOWLEDGMENTS

IN MEDICINE, ROLE MODELS are everything, and while I have had countless mentors who have made lasting impressions on me, I would like to single out three in particular: Dr. Steve Z. Miller, Dr. Glenda Garvey, and Dr. Ingrid Fitz-James. Every single day, I remember what you taught me, and whatever good I have accomplished as a doctor has simply been from doing exactly what you told me to.

Thank you to my parents, who grudgingly conceded that medical school might be a good idea, and to my sisters, for making me feel like I'd made a good decision by following right behind me. I love you guys.

I owe a huge debt of gratitude to my agent, Sharon Bowers, who suggested I write this book in the first place, and to Emily Griffin, for the inglorious task of editing my often convoluted writing and dragging the final product out of me. You both are amazing.

And finally, thank you to my husband, Joe, and my beautiful boys, Cal and Mack. The three of you are my reason for everything, and I love you.

ABOUT THE AUTHOR

MICHELLE AU, MD, is an attending physician of anesthesiology at St. Joseph's Hospital in Atlanta, Georgia. She graduated magna cum laude from Wellesley College in 1999, where for three years she was a weekly humor columnist and cartoonist with the *Wellesley News.* Michelle received her MD from the Columbia University College of Physicians and Surgeons in 2003 and completed a residency in Anesthesiology in 2008.

For the past ten years, she has been writing online about her experiences growing up in the world of academic medicine, as well as the world outside it. The writings from her blog "The Underwear Drawer" (www.theunderweardrawer.blogspot.com) have been featured on WebMD, The Student Doctor Network, Metafilter, and Revolution Health, and her medical comic strips have been featured extensively at dozens of academic medical centers internationally.

She is married to Dr. Joseph Walrath, with whom she has two sons, Cal and Mack, and lives in Atlanta.

323